AF823796

The Palgrave Lacan Series

Series Editors
Calum Neill
Edinburgh Napier University
Edinburgh, UK

Derek Hook
Duquesne University
Pittsburgh, USA

Jacques Lacan is one of the most important and influential thinkers of the 20th century. The reach of this influence continues to grow as we settle into the 21st century, the resonance of Lacan's thought arguably only beginning now to be properly felt, both in terms of its application to clinical matters and in its application to a range of human activities and interests. The Palgrave Lacan Series is a book series for the best new writing in the Lacanian field, giving voice to the leading writers of a new generation of Lacanian thought. The series will comprise original monographs and thematic, multi-authored collections. The books in the series will explore aspects of Lacan's theory from new perspectives and with original insights. There will be books focused on particular areas of or issues in clinical work. There will be books focused on applying Lacanian theory to areas and issues beyond the clinic, to matters of society, politics, the arts and culture. Each book, whatever its particular concern, will work to expand our understanding of Lacan's theory and its value in the 21st century.

Leslie Chapman

Traumatic Neurosis Revisited

Drive-jouissance and the Wounds of Life

palgrave
macmillan

Leslie Chapman
Aldershot, UK

ISSN 2946-4196 ISSN 2946-420X (electronic)
The Palgrave Lacan Series
ISBN 978-3-031-89157-1 ISBN 978-3-031-89158-8 (eBook)
https://doi.org/10.1007/978-3-031-89158-8

© The Editor(s) (if applicable) and The Author(s), under exclusive license to Springer Nature Switzerland AG 2025

This work is subject to copyright. All rights are solely and exclusively licensed by the Publisher, whether the whole or part of the material is concerned, specifically the rights of translation, reprinting, reuse of illustrations, recitation, broadcasting, reproduction on microfilms or in any other physical way, and transmission or information storage and retrieval, electronic adaptation, computer software, or by similar or dissimilar methodology now known or hereafter developed.
The use of general descriptive names, registered names, trademarks, service marks, etc. in this publication does not imply, even in the absence of a specific statement, that such names are exempt from the relevant protective laws and regulations and therefore free for general use.
The publisher, the authors and the editors are safe to assume that the advice and information in this book are believed to be true and accurate at the date of publication. Neither the publisher nor the authors or the editors give a warranty, expressed or implied, with respect to the material contained herein or for any errors or omissions that may have been made. The publisher remains neutral with regard to jurisdictional claims in published maps and institutional affiliations.

Cover illustration: SEAN GLADWELL

This Palgrave Macmillan imprint is published by the registered company Springer Nature Switzerland AG.
The registered company address is: Gewerbestrasse 11, 6330 Cham, Switzerland

If disposing of this product, please recycle the paper.

This book is dedicated to my late and beloved parents, Arthur and Rosemary.

Preface

This book is an attempt to address a question that has puzzled me for many years, although, like many such questions, there is another one that lurks behind it. Having already worked in the mental health field for a number of years prior to commencing my clinical training in the late 1990s, I was well aware of the impact of 'life traumas' on peoples' lives, including sexual violence, poverty and racism, just to mention a few examples. And I deliberately use these three examples because I want to emphasise that such experiences are all 'traumatic' in the sense of psychically *wounding* the subject, which is why in this text I have opted for the term 'wounds of life' as opposed to 'life traumas', 'traumatic events' or something similar.

However, upon entering the world of Lacanian psychoanalysis I became aware of another type of trauma, one which seemed to have very little to do with such 'life-wounds'. This was the idea that the human being's entry into *language* was 'traumatic' in itself. Furthermore, it seemed as if such a 'traumatisation' was a *one-off* event; that is, once the human being had been born into language, and in the process become constituted as a subject (at least in the case of the neurotic subject), then that was it. Similarly, if such a 'traumatic' constitution of the subject failed, as in the case of psychosis, that was it too. In other words, upon being born (or to use a more Heideggerian term, *thrown*) into language, one either was traumatised and became neurotic or was not and thus became psychotic.

Now, clearly, this is somewhat of a parody of a particular reading of Lacan (one which in this book I describe as 'Saussurian'), but like all parodies it contains certain elements of truth and poses a number of difficulties. And the particular difficulty that interests me in this work is how the idea of such an 'inaugural trauma', which seems a very apt way of describing the human being's entry into language, relates to the idea of 'life traumas' or 'wounds of life'. To put it somewhat simplistically, if someone is always already traumatised by virtue of their entry into language, how do they then become *further* traumatised by virtue of exposure to particular life experiences? And just in case this seems a rather abstract question, in my own clinical work I have encountered a number of people who have undergone a range of experiences which would (outside of the Lacanian clinic at least) be described as 'traumatic', ones ranging from sexual violence and abuse to road traffic accidents. And in all these cases I found I was struggling to relate the complexities and nuances of Lacanian theory to the lived suffering in front of me.

This book is essentially an attempt to address (if not answer) this question, this struggle. And I have chosen to use Freud's theory of the traumatic neuroses as a conceptual framework to help me do this. In fact, in the book I refer to this theory as a 'conceptual bridge' between the Lacanian idea of an 'inaugural trauma' and the idea of 'life traumas' or 'wounds of life'. My rationale for adopting this particular theory of Freud and why I think it can act as a 'conceptual bridge' will, I hope, become clear as the book progresses.

However, and this relates to the second question that I referred to at the beginning, this book is also an attempt to construct a re-reading, or perhaps even better, a *re-working,* of Lacan. Before commenting on that, however, I think it is important to note that there is a great deal of *Freud* in this work. This is hardly surprising, perhaps, given the subject matter, but it is also, I think, both a legacy of my own analysis and the fact I have always found Freud's work (albeit in its English translation) extraordinarily deep and incredibly rich in content. As I note in the Introduction, nowadays Freud's work is quite marginalised within the field of 'trauma studies' and in the clinic of trauma. There are a number of reasons to this, some of which I touch upon in the book. In my view, such a marginalisation of Freud is a grave error, both theoretically and clinically; and if nothing else, I hope this work will go some way to 'rehabilitating' Freud within the field of trauma.

There is also quite a bit of Jean Laplanche in this book, which may surprise some Lacanian 'purists' for whom Laplanche, one of a number of Lacan's 'wayward sons', seems nowadays to be pretty much *persona non grata*. The reason for this (which I touch upon briefly in the Introduction) seems to be mainly to do with the fractious politics that characterises psychoanalysis in general and Lacanian psychoanalysis in particular, but as far as Laplanche goes it seems unfortunate. In terms of a re-working of Lacan, and especially within the context of the subject matter of this work, I think there is great deal that Laplanche can bring to the table. So, if this book can contribute towards a rehabilitation of Laplanche as well as that of Freud, then this will be an added bonus.

And yet there is, needless to say, a great deal of Lacan and Lacanian theory in this book, and this brings me back to my 're-working' of Lacan. To give flavour of what this means in practice, I would like to briefly refer to Chap. 3 where, amongst other things, I discuss the influence of psychophysics on Freud's thinking with regard to the operation of the pleasure principle and the principle of constancy. In *Seminar II*, which I go on to discuss in that chapter, Lacan draws upon Freud's ideas in relation to psychophysics (which he refers to as 'energetics') and uses them to develop his own approach to these two principles, and, furthermore, to develop a theory of the drive and of language itself. Essentially, I would argue, he 'substitutes' a theory of cybernetics for that of psychophysics/energetics. This might come as yet another surprise to some readers and especially those who have always associated Lacan's work with his reading of Saussurian semiotics. However, my argument is that Lacan is no Saussurian, even when it comes to his theory of language; in fact, such a theory, along with his reading of Freud's drive theory, is rooted far more in an updated version of Freudian energetics, that is, in the cybernetic theory that was so prevalent in the 1950s and which is now even more prevalent in the guise of artificial intelligence and artificial life. And in case some readers think that I am reverting to some form of Freudian 'biologism', I would just like to remind them of what Lacan said about

Freud's 'biology' as having nothing to do with biology as we would nowadays understand it. In other words, there is nothing 'biological' about Freud's energetics, any more than there is anything of computer science (for example, viewing the human subject as an information processing machine) in Lacan's cybernetics.

What I'm attempting to do in my 're-working' of Lacan is to highlight particular aspects of his work (in the above example his use of cybernetic theory) that have in many writings tended to have been neglected or understated in the wider Lacanian literature, but which, in my view, can be helpful in a 'revisiting' of traumatic neurosis. Another example is my focus on his *Science and Truth* paper as the basis for developing a theory of the Lacanian subject and, going beyond Lacan himself, my references to Miller's concept of 'Lacanian biology' and his idea of jouissance One. In other words, I am not attempting to develop new 'Lacanian' ideas per se; rather, I am drawing upon existing Lacanian theory and reworking it in a particular fashion.

And this leads me to another aspect of my re-working of Lacan: the question of so-called 'French theory' which I discuss in some detail in Chap. 3. As I argue in that chapter, there is nothing particularly 'French' about French theory. Rather, it is a product of the North American academy which has been exported back to Europe; and in the process, I would argue, something vital (in both senses of the word) has been lost. One of the (many) criticisms of Lacanian theory in particular and 'French theory' in general is that this type of thinking is both totally abstract and devoid of any relevance to real-life problems and is completely self-indulgent; in fact, the term one of my students used to describe it to me when I was a university lecturer in the 1990s was 'intellectual masturbation'. In my view this has nothing to do with Lacan's ideas nor, indeed, with those of any other 'French theorist'. Rather, it is the result of a certain type of 'translation' (both linguistic and conceptual) which has severely blunted the subversive and radical edge of these types of ideas. Ironically, perhaps, this seems to mirror the fate of Freud's ideas when they made the trans-Atlantic crossing in the opposite direction and the consequences of which Lacan fought against all of his life.

I will leave it up to the reader to decide whether my re-working of Lacan within the field of trauma has managed to avoid succumbing to the dangers I have just outlined...

Aldershot, UK Leslie Chapman

Acknowledgements

As this book is essentially an amended version of my PhD dissertation I would first like to thank Scott Wilson, who was originally my main supervisor at Kingston University and who then very kindly agreed to continue on an external basis. I always found his input, based on an in-depth knowledge of Lacanian theory, very helpful, albeit at times quite challenging. I would also like to thank Peter Hallward, from the Centre for Research in Modern European Philosophy (CRMEP) at Kingston, who was my main supervisor in the latter part of my research and a great support to me, and who also coined the term 'inaugural trauma' that I use extensively in this work. Thanks also go out to all my past and present colleagues and patients within the psychoanalytic community who, in different ways, have been influential in motivating me to undertake this work. And finally, I would like to thank my wife Maureen, who not only did a sterling job in proofreading the manuscript, but who has always encouraged me to continue, even when I was struggling.

Contents

About the Author

Dr Leslie Chapman is a psychoanalyst working within the Lacanian tradition, based in Hampshire, UK. His analytic formation began at the Centre for Freudian Analysis and Research (CFAR) where he was an Associate Member between 2005 and 2018. He completed his doctoral thesis in 2023 on the topic of the traumatic neuroses and their relation to Lacanian and Freudian theory. Both his clinical and theoretical interests are focused on trauma and its relation to the Lacanian Real. He is particularly interested in how psychoanalysis can challenge the dominant 'mental health' paradigm that sees trauma as something purely 'external' to the individual and which ignores its subjective dimension. More recently, and especially in the light of the conflicts in Ukraine and the Middle East, he has become increasingly focused on the relationship between war and trauma, including the traumatic legacy of past conflicts. He also has a great interest in the opportunities and threats posed by the incursion of artificial intelligence (AI) into the domain of psychoanalysis and the broader talking therapies field. He has written extensively on these topics, both on his own blog and in professional publications.

1

Introduction: An Empire of Trauma?

My central thesis in this book is that Freud's theory of the traumatic neuroses provides a 'conceptual bridge' between the idea that psychical trauma originates in the external word in the form of the 'traumatic event' and the Lacanian idea that the human subject is a product of the traumatising effects of the signifier, brought about by the human being's entry into language. This is based on a particular reading of Freud's theory which draws upon the work of Freud himself, Jacques Lacan, Jacques-Alain Miller, Jean Laplanche, and others. Such a conceptual bridge is necessary, I argue, because (i) it is by no means obvious that these two 'modes' of trauma are related and (ii) showing that there is a relationship between them provides a challenge to the prevailing discourse of trauma which is exemplified in the diagnostic category of post-traumatic stress disorder (PTSD).

Outline of the Argument

The 'popular' view of trauma could perhaps be best summarised as follows:

© The Author(s), under exclusive license to Springer Nature Switzerland AG 2025

L. Chapman, *Traumatic Neurosis Revisited*, The Palgrave Lacan Series,
https://doi.org/10.1007/978-3-031-89158-8_1

> Bad things happen to people at some point(s) in their history and they spend the rest of their lives living with the consequences and trying to come to terms with what happened.

And broadly speaking, this is a view shared by most psychotherapists and other 'trauma specialists', including academics and those in the health and social care professions. Such 'bad things' are usually referred to as 'traumatic events', whilst 'living with the consequences' can include suffering from a range of psychopathological disorders, for example, PTSD, and, on a more collective level, oppression and inequality. 'Coming to terms with' can include working through past traumas in therapy and/or taking a more political stance by trying to address the structural causes of the trauma, for example racism and sexism.

Although Freud could be credited with establishing the concept of psychological trauma in the popular mind, over the last forty years or so, the psychoanalytic model of trauma has been largely rejected, both in the clinic of trauma and increasingly in academia. Instead, from a clinical perspective in particular, the focus is on the role of cognition and neurobiology in the development of psychopathology. And the introduction of the diagnostic category of post-traumatic stress disorder (PTSD) in 1980 has probably done more than anything else to 'legitimise' the idea that trauma can happen to anyone and that, in a sense, 'we are all trauma victims now'. At the same time there has been an increasing focus on the social and cultural dimensions of trauma, and the idea that whole communities can become traumatised. This has led to the development of a body of work that is best described as 'trauma studies'.

The Lacanian approach to trauma is somewhat different and the focus tends to be on the role of language in the formation of the subject. Many Lacanians argue that the subject's entry into language is 'traumatic' and, in fact, is what 'inaugurates' or 'founds' the subject in the first place. If this is indeed the case then it is not clear how 'external' events could further 'traumatise' the subject. In other words, it might seem that 'traumatic events' (or, as I prefer to call them, 'wounds of life') have very little to do with the traumatic effects of the signifier. Even if someone were to visit a psychoanalyst after a 'traumatic experience', for example being involved in a sexual assault or a terrorist attack, it is by no means clear how such an individual would benefit from an analysis as opposed to, say, trauma therapy. However, this seems to set up some form of 'dualism' of trauma whereby the subject is constituted by the trauma of the signifier whilst at the same time being subjected to various 'life traumas'.

One of the key arguments in this book is to show that such a 'dualism' is unnecessary because such 'life traumas' are, in fact, the effects of surplus jouissance, which can be articulated in terms of the operation of the signifier and the circuit of the drive and which in this work I describe as *drive-jouissance*. The critical point here is that such traumatic effects are precisely those that constitute the subject, because such a 'constitution' is not a 'one-off' event but an effect of the continuous impact of the signifier on the subject. However, in 'normal' circumstances such effects are not (consciously) experienced by the subject as traumatic, because the operation of the pleasure principle, or, in Lacanian parlance, the operation of language, functions to regulate jouissance, which can also be conceptualised as a process of deciphering.

This brings us back to Freud and especially his theory of the traumatic neuroses. Freud argues that there are occasions when the psychical apparatus is so overwhelmed by excessive excitations (stimuli) from the outside world that the pleasure principle, which functions to regulate such excitations, is put out of action. This in turn produces a traumatic neurosis. Examples include war, sexual violence, natural disasters and a range of accidents involving various forms of transportation.[1] At first reading Freud's theory appears to be simply another way of describing PTSD, insofar as certain events overwhelm the subject and produce a range of pathological symptoms; and, indeed, this is how some authors have interpreted his theory. However, my argument is that what Freud is describing here is precisely the effects of drive-jouissance upon the subject.

One important point to note at this stage is that my approach to Lacan's theory of language draws upon his ideas in *Seminar II* that utilised the concepts of cybernetics, game and information theory that were

[1] Freud made a number of references to railway accidents in this context.

influential at the time. I argue that such ideas can be used as the basis for a 'cybernetic' reading of Lacan that views language in terms of a regulating 'machine' which functions to decipher jouissance. Such a reading, I argue in later chapters, can be useful in helping to theorise the precise 'mechanisms' by which the subject becomes 'inaugurated' by language, and also raises questions regarding the more 'Saussurian' readings of Lacan in relation to this topic; for example, that the 'traumatic' effects of language are primarily based around (Symbolic) castration.

The other key element of my argument relates to Freud's concept of *Nachträglichkeit*. This is the idea that trauma is only ever constructed retroactively, often much later on in the life of the subject. This is important for several reasons: firstly, it calls into question the idea of an 'original trauma', or, more precisely, an 'original (traumatic) event'; secondly, it is an idea utilised by Lacan in order to explain the retroactive nature of both meaning and the drive, which are crucial when it comes to the question of the deciphering of jouissance. And thirdly, it raises important questions regarding the relationship between trauma, temporality and history.

An Empire of Trauma?

> Sometimes trauma seems to be everywhere. Nearly any minor setback can be casually described as "traumatic", to the point that the term risks becoming useless. It is trivialized by being employed to refer to inconsequential, ultimately harmless niggles in our daily lives. Yet trauma is also real. To deny it risks perpetuating it. Victims, survivors and witnesses of traumatic experiences, as well as those who feel themselves somehow to have been affected or implicated by them, have wanted to talk and write about trauma, and to become involved in other cultural forms of remembrance and testimony.[2]

[2] Hanna Meretoja and Colin Davis, 'Introduction to Literary Trauma Studies', in *The Routledge Companion to Literature and Trauma*, ed. by Hanna Meretoja and Colin Davis (Milton: Taylor and Francis, 2020), 1–8.

These remarks by Hanna Meretoja and Colin Davis neatly encapsulate one of the key dilemmas regarding trauma: on the one hand trauma does indeed seem to be everywhere as more and more everyday experiences become, or are at risk of becoming, 'traumatic'. On the other hand, it seems difficult to deny that there is a reality to trauma and that at least some experiences deserve to be described in such terms. But even here there are difficulties because it is by no means clear in the literature of trauma what the term actually means in the first place. This is especially so, I argue, when it comes to the term 'traumatic event, which I will have more to say about later on in this Introduction.

Despite all these difficulties, the concept of trauma appears to be firmly implanted in mainstream social discourse. And, as I will argue shortly, a great deal of this has to do with the 'legitimation' of trauma brought about by the 'invention' of PTSD in the 1980s. Trauma is now a dominant force, at least in Western societies; in fact, Didier Fassin and Richard Rechtman have even gone so far as to speak of the *empire* of trauma.[3] Nicole Sütterlin has noted that the concept of psychological trauma is often portrayed as a product of *modernity*, although she is also at pains to point out that this view is itself now being contested and there is growing interest in the 'pre-modern' genealogy of trauma.[4] She gives the examples of the pedagogical work of Johann Heinrich Campe, the empirical psychology of Karl-Philipp Moritz, Johann Christian Reil's neurophysiology and the idealist philosophy of Johann Gottlieb Fichte, all working in the late eighteenth and early nineteenth century and who all helped develop the idea of the modern subject as inherently *vulnerable*. Sütterlin goes on to argue that:

> In the literary texts of authors such as Johann Wolfgang Goethe, Clemens Brentano and E.T.A. Hoffmann, this notion of vulnerability as the foundation of the modern self gives rise to depictions of what later would be called trauma. Not only do they provide remarkably accurate descriptions of

[3] Didier Fassin and Richard Rechtman, *The Empire of Trauma: An Inquiry into the Condition of Victimhood* (Princeton: Princeton University Press, 2009).

[4] Nicole A. Sütterlin, 'History of Trauma Theory', in *The Routledge Companion to Literature and Trauma*, ed. by Hanna Meretoja and Colin Davis (Milton: Taylor and Francis, 2020), 11–22.

> symptoms which today are associated with PTSD, but they connect these features with specific traumatic events such as physical or sexual assault in childhood. In developing this aetiology, they appear (sic) were one step ahead of the burgeoning psychiatry of their time.[5]

And perhaps the idea of the *vulnerable subject* is key to understanding the ever-growing domination of trauma's empire. The sub-title of Fassin and Rechtman's book hints at this too ('An Inquiry into the Condition of Victimhood'), although the concept of victimhood is not necessarily, I would argue, equivalent to that of the vulnerable subject; being vulnerable would appear to be more of an existential condition, whereas seeing oneself as a 'victim' would appear to be a particular way of reflecting upon such a condition. One of the central arguments in this book, following Freud, is that all subjects are 'vulnerable' in terms of being exposed to the 'wounds of life' (I will explain this terminology shortly). Furthermore, I will be focusing on a particular incarnation of the 'vulnerable' subject, that is, the subject of modern science, which, according to Lacan, is also the subject of psychoanalysis (and trauma).

In terms of the colonising effects of trauma's empire (to pursue Fassin and Rechtman's metaphor), there is perhaps no better example than the near universal acceptance (at least within the discourse of Western psychiatry and clinical psychology) of the diagnostic category of PTSD. According to the standard narrative of psychological trauma, before PTSD there were a range of psychological 'conditions' or 'disorders' that were essentially describing the same set of symptoms, which included nightmares, flashbacks, panic attacks, depression, anxiety, difficulties in concentrating, and so on. Much of this narrative focuses on how such symptoms manifested themselves in war, starting with the Great War, which began in 1914, and, depending on which country you were living in at the time, may or may not have ended in 1918.[6]

As a number of authors have argued, PTSD is a direct legacy of the Vietnam War (as opposed to the Great one) and of intense political lobbying by a group of therapists, psychiatrists, and veterans. In 1980 the

[5] *Ibid.*, 15.

[6] For many in Eastern Europe, the War certainly did not end on 11 November 1918. Instead, the 'official' end of hostilities ushered in years of civil war.

term PTSD was finally recognised as a psychiatric category and took its place in the third edition of the Diagnostic and Statistical Manual of Mental Disorders (DSM-III), the 'bible' of the American psychiatric profession.[7] At the same time though, there are striking similarities with the Great War. Like its predecessor, the Vietnam War was (and still is) subjected to a process of 'reimagining', to paraphrase the title of Samuel Hynes' study of the Great War and of English culture.[8] And many of the same issues were at stake in what might be described as 'Generation Love meets Generation (Cold) War'. There was the question of continuity versus discontinuity: that is, was the war really a major turning point for the United States or was it simply the continuation of a long, drawn-out historical process? Was it *a generational* war, of young versus old? Was it a question of 'culture versus *Kultur*', the progressive, enlightened liberal left versus the old, reactionary, and philistine right? All these questions had been rehearsed (though not, as it turns out, resolved) in the 1920s.

And in the middle of this there is the question of trauma. What to make of, and what to do with, all those psychologically damaged individuals who came back from the war:

> More than any other war in the twentieth century, Vietnam redefined the social role of psychiatry and society's perspective of mental health. Five years after the fall of Saigon, a new psychiatric term was devised, tailored to the needs of veterans. Psychiatric counselling was made available on an unparalleled scale, paid for by the United States government. Even more significantly, Vietnam helped to create a new 'consciousness of trauma' in Western society.[9]

Ben Shephard, whom I have just quoted, argues that there were four key elements that lay behind this new 'consciousness of trauma', and the

---

[7] For a very readable account of the political and psychiatric 'construction' of PTSD, as well as its various 'predecessors', I would recommend Ben Shephard's *War of Nerves* (London: Jonathan Cape, 2000) and also Wilbur Scott's 'PTSD in DSM-III: A Case in the Politics of Diagnosis and Disease', *Social Problems*, 37.3 (1990), 294–310. Fassin and Rechtman cover much of the same ground in the work already cited.

[8] Samuel Hynes, *A War Imagined: The First World War and English Culture* (London: The Bodley Head Ltd., 1990).

[9] Ben Shephard, *A War of Nerves* (London: Jonathan Cape, 2000).

appearance of this 'new psychiatric term' (PTSD). The first was the 'acrid' political aftermath of the war in the United States. This was the era of Watergate and where the government itself was on trial. Vietnam, as the war that the US lost, was a toxic and divisive subject, and the question of how it had affected individual (US) combatants was itself a contentious subject. Those who opposed the war wanted to emphasise the negative psychological effects, whilst those who had supported the war wanted to play down such effects. It should also be remembered that, unlike the Second World War, there was no heroic homecoming for soldiers; rather they were more likely to be treated with suspicion and contempt.

The second element was the legacy of the Nazi Holocaust, and to a lesser extent, that of Hiroshima and Nagasaki. As survivors of the concentration camps started to come forward in large numbers in the 1970s to tell their stories, there was a growing realisation amongst American psychiatrists and other mental health professionals of the traumas that the camp inmates had experienced, and in many cases were still experiencing. Some professionals started to make the connection with the experiences of Vietnam veterans and even coined the term 'survivor syndrome'. This also contributed to a gradual broadening of the notion of trauma, which until then had been confined to the experiences of soldiers in combat.

The third element was the biological revolution in American psychiatry, and with it the growing use of psychotropic drugs to treat a wide range of mental health problems. This was reflected in the proposals for the third edition of the DSM. The two previous versions (DSM I and DSM II) had been heavily influenced by psychoanalytic ideas and terminology, and, perhaps even more significantly in relation to the concerns of the Vietnam veterans, both previous versions had included a category for war-related trauma. In DSM III, however, there was to be no separate classification for trauma, because it was being argued that existing psychiatric categories were adequate to explain the problems suffered by combatants and veterans. This had serious implications for veterans, because in order to receive proper support they felt they needed a separate 'war trauma' category; and, furthermore, with regard to possible financial compensation, claimants needed to show a link between combat experiences and their subsequent psychological trauma.

This brings us to the fourth, and perhaps most crucial element of all: the politics of the Vietnam veterans, and particularly their forging of alliances with sympathetic psychiatrists and psychotherapists. Some veteran organisations started to use the media to highlight the psychological effects of the war, and a number of 'vet horror stories' appeared, portraying deeply disturbed, and often heavily armed, ex-combatants running amok in the towns and cities of America. Inevitably, perhaps, this was picked up by Hollywood, and films such as *Taxi Driver* and *Rambo* helped reinforce the perception that the war had seriously traumatised a whole generation of young Americans, even though the statistics did not back this up.

However, the real breakthrough came when psychiatrists sympathetic to the veterans' cause started to develop a more robust theoretical foundation for trauma, and one of the key individuals here was Mardi Horowitz. He argued that whenever a person experiences a stressful life event (his term for a traumatic experience), they go through a particular process, which is comprised of specific phases: (1) Outcry, (2) Denial, (3) Intrusiveness, (4) Working through, (5) Completion.[10] One of the key points about Horowitz's theory is that it acknowledges that individual predisposition or pre-existing psychopathology may play a role in trauma. This is because he argues that some individuals are unable to 'work through' or 'process' the initial experience. And the reason for this, according to Horowitz, is that some individuals have a more 'brittle' or 'unstable' self-concept or cognitive schema regarding their levels of competence; in other words, some individuals are prone to regard themselves as 'incompetent', 'defective' and 'worthless'. This means that when such individuals are exposed to a stressful life-event their feelings of negative self-worth are likely to impact negatively on their ability to work-through the memory of the event.

Perhaps more importantly, though, the work of Horowitz and his colleagues was critical in creating a 'bridge' between war-related trauma and trauma experienced by individuals in non-combat situations. In other words, it is no longer just war or conflict that is traumatic, but life itself.

[10] Mardi J. Horowitz, "Post Traumatic Stress Disorders," *Behavioral Sciences & the Law* 1, no. 3 (1983): 9–23.

In practical, psychiatric terms, the immediate effect was the creation of post-traumatic stress disorder and its inclusion in DSM III in 1980, where it has remained ever since, and can now be found in DSM-5.[11] The longer-lasting impact, as Shephard points out, is that the whole cultural perception of trauma changed, and 'life-trauma' essentially became 'legitimated' in public discourse.

Earlier I briefly touched upon the idea of the 'vulnerable subject' and argued that this does not necessarily equate with the idea of 'victimhood'. However, over recent decades there has been a steady movement towards the idea of trauma sufferers as victims, which is a process that Nadia Abu El-Haj explores in some detail in her book *Combat Trauma*.[12] El-Haj's starting point is the Vietnam War and the emergence of 'Post-Vietnam Syndrome' (the immediate precursor to PTSD) in the 1970s. What is particularly interesting, in my view, is her idea of a shift from *perpetrator* to *victim*, which was completed in the wake of the 9/11 bombings and the subsequent 'war on terror' (that then morphed into the wars in Iraq and Afghanistan). For example, the very same individuals who had perpetrated atrocities in Vietnam (the My Lai massacre being only one of many) had, by the 1980s, become recast as victims of the war. El-Haj explains that:

> The combat-trauma imaginary of the new millennium emerges from a particular reading of the (Vietnam) war and what is presumed to be its major lesson—that the mistreatment of US veterans by a hostile anti-war public upon their return from the battlefields of Vietnam must never be repeated … while during the war and in its immediate aftermath a pervasive political critique of the war and US military brutality on the battlefields was shared across diverse swaths of American society, a decade hence, the war had been transformed into an "American tragedy" and the critique redirected from US militarism as such onto the American public. In the words of one historian, "the deepest shame related to the Vietnam war" became "not the war itself, but America's failure to embrace its military veterans."[13]

[11] Please note: Arabic numerals replaced Roman ones in DSM-5.

[12] Nadia Abu El-Haj, *Combat Trauma: Imaginaries of War and Citizenship in Post-9/11 America (Kindle Edition)* (London: Verso, 2002).

[13] *Ibid.*, 46.

But where does psychoanalysis fit into this? Although, as Sütterlin reminds us, Freud did not invent the concept of psychical trauma, he probably did more than any theoretician or clinician to lay the foundations for its 'imperial' status in present day cultural discourse. This is somewhat ironic, because at the very moment trauma became 'accepted' and 'mainstream', Freud's ideas were rapidly being displaced by cognitive and neurobiological approaches to trauma. And part of the reason for this appears to be a fundamental misunderstanding of the way Freud's views changed on the subject, and especially his idea regarding 'childhood seduction'. According to Sütterlin: "Today, Freud is often discredited for abandoning the notion of real trauma as a pathological determinant and subsuming it into a model of intrapsychic conflicts."[14] And El-Haj makes the important point that, to be taken seriously, the 'victims' of trauma need traumatic events which are 'literal' rather than the result of psychical construction and whose 'actuality' could be called into question. As she notes, this applies particularly to the *memory* of traumatic events:

> For those advocating on behalf of victims of sexual assault, rendering traumatic *memory* literal likewise served crucial forensic purposes. Sexual assault victims' memories needed to be accurate, not just credible if fathers, boyfriends, acquaintances, and even strangers were going to be prosecuted for the crimes of incest and rape. This battle was waged not only against existing psychiatric practice, or even just against a particular social and political imaginary, but also against a judicial environment in which refusing to believe and/or blaming the victim was the norm.[15]

As I will argue in the next chapter (and, at various points, throughout this work) Freud's 'abandonment' of his theory of childhood seduction is something of a misnomer. In fact, I would argue that his concept of the traumatic neuroses, which he retained throughout his work, is proof of this. In my view, it was not so much an 'abandonment' but, rather, an *augmentation*. Put simply, he did not simply give up on his earlier (pre-1897) idea that the roots of his patients' neuroses lay in infantile

---

[14] Sütterlin, 'History of Trauma Theory', 13.

[15] *Ibid.*, 91, italic in original.

sexual experiences, but rather recognised the key role of fantasy, repression and the broader process of psychical working over that took place for each of his patients.

Lacan's position regarding trauma is more complex. On the one hand he argues in *Seminar XI*[16] that trauma is a manifestation of the Real and is linked to Aristotle's concept of *tuché* (chance). On the other hand, precisely because of this relationship between trauma and the Real,[17] I would argue that Lacan tends to 'downplay' the former concept in his work; in other words, Lacan's theory of the Real effectively 'absorbs' his theory of trauma. In this present work I do not have the space to elaborate Lacan's approach to the Real;[18] however, with regards to my central thesis, the Real has a particular prominence with regards to the formation of the human subject, which Lacan argues is both the subject of science and the subject of psychoanalysis. As I argue in Chap. 4, the subject of science is, in effect, a 'dual' subject; on the one hand it is the subject of the Real which is excluded from language, whilst on the other hand it is a 'sutured' subject, a 'stand-in' for the occluded subject (of the Real). The Real is also closely linked to the concepts of jouissance and the object *a*, which in his later work Lacan will refer to as surplus jouissance and as a 'piece of the Real'. And the endless repetition of the drive and its production of jouissance is in the domain of the Real, which in 'normal' circumstances is regulated by language—which is how Lacan conceptualised Freud's pleasure principle.

The work of Lacan's son-in-law, Jacques-Alain Miller, features quite prominently in this work, especially with regards to his development of the concept of suture, which I referred to above, and his 'six paradigms of jouissance', which provide a useful framework for discussing Lacan's

[16] Jacques Lacan, *The Four Fundamental Concepts of Psycho-Analysis* (London: Penguin, 1979) (Hereafter *Seminar XI*).

[17] Please note that Lacan uses the terms 'Real' and 'real' interchangeably in different parts of his teaching, as does Jacques-Alain Miller. For the sake of consistency I will stick to using the uppercase version ('Real') throughout this work.

[18] For an excellent introduction to this topic I would recommend Tom Eyers' *Lacan and the Concept of the 'Real'* (Basingstoke, Hampshire: Palgrave Macmillan, 2012) in which he develops a materialist theory of the Real. Lacan's *Seminar XXIII* (Cambridge: Polity Press, 2016) is also useful because here he develops his 'last' theory of the three registers (Real, Symbolic and Imaginary) utilising the theory of the Borromean knot.

development of the idea of jouissance and its relation to the drive and the object *a*. Miller is a key figure in the more recent history of psychoanalysis, not least because of his founding of the World Association of Psychoanalysis in 1992. He is also one of the main driving forces behind the so-called 'later Lacan', which focuses on Lacan's work in the 1970s.[19]

In this book I also draw upon work of Jean Laplanche, who was both an analysand of Lacan's and, during the 1950s, a regular attendee at his seminars. However, Lacan and Laplanche began to part ways when Laplanche and Serge Leclaire gave a paper on the unconscious at the Bonneval Congress in 1960 which Lacan took exception to. In spite of this, Laplanche claimed to retain "a great deal of affection' for Lacan and in an interview in 1990 stated that: "He only ever did me good, so I have no personal grievance to bear towards him.[20] It would seem, however, that such affection was not reciprocated, and Laplanche's name very rarely features in Lacanian literature. This is perhaps just one example of the fractious relationships that have been rife within the Lacanian field since Lacan's 'excommunication' from the International Psychoanalytic Association (IPA) in 1964. This wasn't helped by the fact that by the late 1960s Lacan, the erstwhile maverick, had become very much the orthodoxy of French psychoanalysis.[21]

Laplanche, by this time, was developing his own approach to psychoanalysis and in many ways it could be seen as his own 'return to Freud', just as Lacan felt he was returning to the truth of Freud's work. In a number of key texts, and especially in *Life and Death in Psychoanalysis*[22] and *New Foundations for Psychoanalysis*[23] Laplanche revisited a number of key Freudian concepts, including the drive, the pleasure principle, the ego,

[19] For a good introduction to the 'later Lacan' see Véronique Voruz and Bogdan Wolf's book of the same name: Véronique Voruz and Bogdan Wolf, eds., *The Later Lacan: An Introduction* (New York: Suny Press, 2007).

[20] Jean Laplanche, 'Interview: Jean Laplanche Talks to Martin Stanton', in *Jean Laplanche: Seduction, Translation and the Drives*, trans. by Martin Stanton (London: Institute of Contemporary Arts, 1992), 4.

[21] For a useful discussion of such 'Lacan wars' see Monique David-Menard and Brian Massumi, 'Lacanians Against Lacan', *Social Text*, 6, 1982, 86–111.

[22] Jean Laplanche, *Life and Death in Psychoanalysis* (Baltimore: John Hopkins University Press, 1985).

[23] Jean Laplanche, *New Foundations for Psychoanalysis* (Oxford: Basil Blackwell, 1989).

and, perhaps more controversially, the idea of childhood sexuality. Laplanche's work is also important because of his detailed examination of Freud's concept of the pleasure principle and some of the contradictions it presents in his work, and his reading of Freud's theory of *Nachträglichkeit,* which I explore at length later on in this text.

Over the last thirty years or so, trauma research has considerably widened its scope and has developed into an academic discipline in its own right, which is often referred to as 'trauma studies'. In terms of the field itself, there is no specific 'definition': rather, it is more the case that a body of work has developed that, to quote Sütterlin again, sees trauma as "…a key interpretative category of our time." She goes onto note that ever since PTSD was introduced into the third edition of the DSM "the concept of psychological trauma has virtually exploded…"[24] Likewise, Fassin and Rechtman argue that: "The idea that tragic and painful events, whether individual or collectively experienced, leave marks in the mind which are then seen as "scars" by analogy to those left on the body, is … easily accepted."[25]

Perhaps one of key characteristics of trauma studies is its *interdisciplinary* scope. Although the modern idea of trauma and the concept of traumatic neurosis originated in the mid-nineteenth century with the advent of rail travel and so-called 'railway spine', whereby those involved in railway accidents presented with physical disorders with no apparent organic injury, the idea of psychological trauma has now reached well beyond the doctor's consulting room. In particular, and to continue with Fassin and Rechtman's imperial metaphor, trauma has 'colonised' literary studies and the social sciences, including history, sociology and cultural studies. The idea that whole societies, as well as groups of individuals within those societies, can become traumatised has now become accepted almost without question, and literature has become seen as an especially powerful medium for exploring and 'deconstructing' such traumas:

> For literary trauma studies, a crucial question concerns the relationship between culture and trauma. While psychology has focused on the psychic

[24] Sütterlin, 'History of Trauma Theory', 11.

[25] Fassin and Rechtman, *The Empire of Trauma*, 4.

> traces left on the individual by a traumatic event, approaches focussing on literature and other creative media are often interested in the cultural and social dimensions of trauma.[26]

Academics such as Jeffery Alexander have also contributed to the field by developing more comprehensive social or cultural models of trauma.[27] These models examine in some detail how trauma and, more specifically, *narratives* of trauma, become constructed by particular groups and disseminated to the wider world. And the concept of the trauma narrative is crucial in both the academic study of trauma and its clinical treatment. Most, if not all, clinical interventions (for example, in the treatment of PTSD) are based around helping the subject give meaning to their experiences (or, more precisely, to the *memories* of such experiences).[28] This is even the case with many psychoanalytically orientated therapies, whereby the subject gradually constructs a history (that is, a personal narrative) of their traumatic past. Such narratives serve not only to give meaning to the subject's apparently meaningless experiences, but also situates them in a wider, social context and essentially gives the subject an *identity*, that is, as a trauma 'victim' or 'survivor'. And this is not only true on an individual level but also at the level of the group, community or society, for example, Holocaust survivors and their descendants.

The problem of giving meaning to apparently meaningless experiences is explored in two of the influential 'founding' texts of contemporary trauma studies. In her book *Unclaimed Experience* Cathy Caruth argues that trauma is a form of experience that cannot be directly articulated (hence its 'unclaimed' nature) but asserts itself retroactively through the process of *Nachträglichkeit* (her term is 'belatedness') in the form of *history*.[29] In other words, history is an attempt to construct a narrative out of the void (what Lacan would call the Real) of lived human experience.

---

[26] Davis and Meretoja, 'Introduction to literary trauma studies', 4.

[27] Jeffrey C Alexander, *Trauma: A Social Theory* (Cambridge: Polity Press, 2012).

[28] For example, cognitive behavioural therapy (CBT). One exception would be eye movement desensitization and reprocessing therapy (EMDR) which relies more on processing traumatic memories at the neurobiological level.

[29] Cathy Caruth, *Unclaimed Experience: Trauma, Narrative and History* (John Hopkins University Press, 1996).

One of the implications here is that history can never, in a Rankean sense, 'tell it as it was'; but, rather, can only ever construct specific accounts of how it might have been. I shall be exploring Caruth's argument in more detail later on.

Shoshana Felman and Dori Laub, on the other hand, in their book *Testimony* ask: "What is the relation between literature, testimony, between the writer and the witness? What is the relation between the act of witnessing and testifying, and the acts of writing and of reading, particularly in our era?"[30] The particular focus of their book is the Holocaust and Holocaust testimony, including a detailed analysis of Claude Lanzmann's film *Shoah*. As Felman notes:

> It (*Shoah*) is a film about witnessing: about the witnessing of a catastrophe. What is testified to is limit-experiences whose overwhelming impact constantly puts to the test the limits of the witness and of witnessing, at the same time that it constantly unsettles and puts into question the very limits of reality.[31]

In the wake of such texts, however, there have been a growing number of critiques of the genre, especially from a post-colonial and decolonising perspective. One of the problems with trauma studies, according to its critics, is that because of its predominately Western European and North American heritage it is essentially imposing a very specific type of trauma discourse onto cultures and societies which do not share its basic assumptions, including those regarding the nature of human subjectivity itself and the nature of trauma. For example, Jessica Murray argues that: "The genesis of trauma theory in Freudian analysis means that these (European rooted) theories have, from their very beginning, been framed in psychoanalytic terms and psychoanalysis is a necessarily individualizing practice."[32] And although, as I argued above, the majority of contemporary theories are *not* psychoanalytically grounded, her basic argument still

[30] Shoshana Felman and Dori Laub, *Testimony: Crises of Witnessing in Literature, Psychoanalysis, and History* (New York: Routledge, 1992), xiii.

[31] *Ibid.*, 205.

[32] Jessica Murray, 'A Post-Colonial and Feminist Reading of Selected Testimonies to Trauma in Post-Liberation South Africa and Zimbabwe', *Journal of African Cultural Studies*, 21.1 (2009), 4.

seems to stand because the dominant cognitive-behavioural and neurobiological theories of trauma are still very much *intra-psychically* focused.

Irene Visser is critical of the idea that history, as portrayed by Caruth and other 'Eurocentric' trauma theorists, lacks factuality; in other words, the idea that history does not describe things that actually happened:

> For instance, the trauma of Māori history as the aftermath of colonialism as depicted in literature by Māori authors such as Witi Ihimaera, Apirana Taylor, and Patricia Grace is not the anti-historical, phylogenetic, and mythic trauma of Freudian theory, but the trauma of concrete historical factuality: of dispossession, of land loss, and of instances of racial discrimination.[33]

And Dovile Budryte reminds us that the 'Eurocentrism' of contemporary trauma studies is predominately *Western* European in her study of the complexity of memory landscapes in post-communist Eastern Europe and the way different groups within that region deal with the traumas of both Nazi and Soviet colonisation and their aftermaths.[34]

'Wounds of Life' or 'Traumatic Events'?

Before outlining the structure of this work, I just wanted to briefly comment upon my use of the term 'wounds of life' in the subtitle. Although there were a number of different possibilities that I could have used, for example, 'life traumas', 'traumatic events', 'traumatic experiences' and so on, I opted for the first term for two reasons. Firstly, the reference to 'wounding' makes sense etymologically. As Laplanche and Pontalis point out, the term trauma (from the Greek *τραῦμα* meaning 'wound') has a long history in medicine and surgery, and refers to a physical injury (generally, but not always, of the skin) and the effects of such an injury on the

[33] Irene Visser, 'Decolonizing Trauma Theory: Retrospect and Prospects', *Humanities*, 4.2 (2015), 254.

[34] Dovile Budryte, 'Decolonization of Trauma and Memory Politics: Insights from Eastern Europe', in *Decolonizing Trauma Studies : Trauma and Postcolonialism*, ed. by Sonya Andermahr, (Switzerland: MDPI - Multidisciplinary Digital Publishing Institute, 2016), 153–68.

organism as a whole.[35] They go on to argue that: "In adopting the term, psycho-analysis carries the three ideas implicit in it over on to the psychical level: the idea of a violent shock, the idea of a wound and the idea of consequences affecting the whole organisation."[36]

As I note in the next chapter, in conceptualising trauma Freud did not utilise the first idea, that is, (psychical) trauma as involving a violent shock, or at least not in any crude sense of the word; instead, he employed the idea of *excess excitation*. However, the metaphor of the 'wound' is certainly there in his work, along with that of the 'breach'. And, with regards to the third idea, that trauma affects the whole psychical apparatus, this is certainly the case with both neurosis and (even more so, perhaps) psychosis. One advantage of this term is that it emphasises the *damaging effects* of certain experiences and the idea of *rupture* or *tear* in the fabric of the subject's reality, which, as I argue in the Conclusion, can be seen as the consequence of an irruption of the Real into such a reality.

The second reason I decided to use the term 'wounds of life' is because the concept of the 'traumatic event' is somewhat problematic in the context of my argument. I shall come back to this in more detail in the Conclusion, but, put briefly, the problem relates to the question of 'externality'. Although there is no intrinsic reason why such events should be 'external' to the subject, this is often how they are portrayed and is very much linked to the question of *victimhood* and the idea that trauma is something that 'happens' to people through no fault of their own. One of the key arguments in this book is that the dichotomy between 'external' and 'internal' is both problematic and unnecessary, and Freud's concept of the traumatic neuroses is a way to 'bridge' such a dichotomy.

The Structure of the Book

Chapter 2 'sets the scene' for the rest of the book by exploring Freud's concept of the traumatic neuroses and some of the key questions it raises. I begin by briefly discussing the broader concept of trauma in Freud's

---

[35] Jean Laplanche and Jean-Bertrand Pontalis, *The Language of Psychoanalysis* (London: Karnac Books, 1988).

[36] *Ibid.*, 466.

work, and especially the idea that although he originally argued that his patients' psychoneuroses were the result of actual childhood sexual experiences, he abandoned this theory in 1897 in favour of a more intrapsychical theory which focused on the operations of the drive, fantasy, repression and the unconscious. My argument here is that the term 'abandonment' is somewhat misleading, and that it is more helpful to think of an *augmentation* of his original theory.

As I argue in the chapter, Freud started using the terms 'traumatic neuroses' (plural) and 'traumatic neurosis' (singular) early on in his work and continued to employ the concept throughout his life. However, it was not until much later on in Freud's work, and particularly in *Beyond the Pleasure Principle* and *Inhibitions, Symptoms and Anxiety*, that he places more emphasis on the idea that 'excitations', both external and internal, are the real cause of trauma.

One of the key examples of the traumatic neuroses, which I discuss in the chapter, is that of the 'war neuroses', which Freud became increasingly interested in in the wake of the Great War when he and some of his colleagues had direct experience of treating soldiers who were exhibiting a range of psychopathological symptoms relating to their experiences in combat. One of the interesting points about the war neuroses was that Freud and his colleagues were using them to *refute* the idea that such neuroses disproved the idea that neuroses were rooted in childhood sexual conflicts. I also critically examine Freud's concept of the *actual neuroses* and propose, contrary to the arguments of Paul Verhaeghe and others, that in his later work Freud essentially abandoned this idea and replaced it with that of the traumatic neuroses.

Because so much of Freud's argument regarding the traumatic neuroses rests on the idea of a disruption of the pleasure principle by excessive excitations, Chap. 3 is devoted to exploring the concept of such a principle in some detail. Freud's basic idea is that the pleasure principle regulates the activity of the psychical apparatus and especially the operation of the drives, which are a constant force and therefore a constant source of excitation. However, things become more complicated in Freud's later writings because in *Beyond the Pleasure Principle* he introduces the idea, linked closely to his concept of the death drive, of a 'tendency towards zero' or the 'zero principle', which is the notion that the organism is always striving towards a state of null excitation, and at one point Freud equates this tendency with the pleasure principle.

Freud's argument becomes even more complex when it comes to the principle of constancy, an idea which Freud 'borrows' from Gustav Fechner, because on the one hand he seems to equate this with the 'tendency towards zero' whilst on the other hand he argues that it is another way to describe the regulatory function of the pleasure principle. And it is this ambiguity regarding the pleasure principle and Freud's conflation of it in parts of his writings with the principle of constancy that I discuss in some detail in the middle part of the chapter, with a particular reference to Laplanche's arguments regarding the death drive and its relation to both the pleasure principle and the principle of constancy. This is in order to try and 'unpick' some of the apparent contradictions in Freud's exposition of this subject matter.

In the latter part of the chapter I explore Lacan's approach to the pleasure principle, which, I argue, marks a shift from a theory of *energetics* (Freud's) to one of *cybernetics*. I illustrate this through a discussion of Lacan's arguments in *Seminar II* where he utilises cybernetic theory to explore how language, especially in the form of a 'binary code', can act both as a self-regulating system whilst at the same time having a disruptive and somewhat paradoxical 'creative-destructive' effect on the human subject. This leads him to develop the more radical idea that the death drive is linked closely to the Symbolic order rather than being some kind of (quasi) biological form of 'entropy' in the psychical apparatus. Within the context of these arguments, and drawing especially upon the work of Lydia Liu, I also examine the influence of 'French Theory' on Lacan's work and how this has shifted the emphasis away from the important legacy of cybernetics and information theory in Lacan's work.

The concept of a cybernetic theory of language and the unconscious lead onto the question of the role of language in the constitution or inauguration of the human subject and how this relates to trauma. This is the focus of Chap. 4 and much of my discussion revolves around Lacan's argument in *Science and Truth* that the subject of psychoanalysis is also the subject of modern science. As I argue in the chapter, Lacan is not suggesting a crude type of 'causal' relationship between the emergence of modern (mathematically based) science and the appearance of a particular type of human subject, which Lacan equates with the Cartesian *cogito*. Rather, he argues that there is a *correlation* between the two and, more crucially, that without the emergence of the subject of science there would be no psychoanalysis. In order to explore the logic of Lacan's argument in this respect I explore in some detail the idea of the Cartesian subject in relation to modern science and also the work of Alexandre Koyré, whose writings were very influential upon Lacan in his understanding of the development of science since the late fifteenth century.

A particularly key idea that I refer to in the chapter is Lacan's use of the concept of *suture*. This only gets a brief mention in *Science and Truth* but, I argue, is critical in understanding the paradoxical nature of the Lacanian subject: on the one hand this is the subject of language and discourse (and more specifically, the subject of the discourse of *science*) and yet on the other hand is an *excluded* subject, the subject of the Real. In order to elucidate this concept I examine in some detail Jacques-Alain Miller's treatment of the topic in a presentation he gave in *Seminar XII* and in a subsequent published text, and which draws extensively on the ideas of the mathematician Gottlob Frege. Lacan also places great emphasis on the idea of truth as cause and in order to follow his reasoning here I explore his use of Aristotle's concepts of *tuché* and *automaton* in Seminar XI, which links closely to his arguments regarding the Real and trauma. My concluding argument in this chapter is that the Lacanian subject *is* trauma, is a subject of the Real, and is essentially an effect of the language of modern science.

Chapter 5 explores the concept of the drive and how it relates to both language and jouissance. The chapter begins with a brief clarification of the term 'drive' (*Treib*), which in Strachey's translation is (mis)rendered as 'instinct', before moving onto a close examination of Freud's drive theory, particularly as he developed it in *Instincts and their Vicissitudes*. The key focus here is the idea of the drive as a 'frontier' or 'boundary' concept and that it can be thought of as having four 'components': pressure, aim, object and source. This allows Freud to argue that the paths to the drive's satisfaction can vary considerably as can its object. I then move onto to discuss Lacan's reading of *Instincts and their Vicissitudes* in *Seminar XI* and especially his idea of the drive as 'montage' and that its 'satisfaction' is a product of its endless circuit around the object *a*, rather than 'obtaining' a specific object. This lays the foundation for the idea that the drive 'produces' jouissance in such an endless circuit.

I then explore Lacan's concept of jouissance within the framework of Miller's 'six paradigms of jouissance', and with a particular focus on paradigms four to six. One of the key points to emerge here is the idea that jouissance became a central part of Lacan's thinking and teaching in his later work, which involved a reworking of his concepts of language and the signifier. Another key idea is that *surplus jouissance*, which is closely linked to the circuit of the drive, and which Miller argues can be thought of as 'crumbs of jouissance'. Such 'crumbs' extend the register of the object *a* to a whole range of objects in the wider world, and, as I argue in the conclusion, form the basis for the proliferation of jouissance (and trauma) in the contemporary world. There is also the critical idea, which Miller discusses in the context of a 'Lacanian biology' and the idea of the 'body event', that jouissance is embodied and that the living body is the condition of jouissance. I conclude by discussing the concept of jouissance in relation to Freud's idea of the traumatic memory, with particular reference to Nestor Braunstein's work on this topic.

In Chap. 6 I focus on one of the problems that any theory of trauma has to contend with, psychoanalytic or otherwise, which is that in many instances the symptoms of trauma can occur many months, years or even decades (and some case centuries) after the 'original' traumatic experience. Freud argued that this was due to a process he called *Nachträglichkeit* which is the idea that trauma is constructed *retroactively.* I explore this idea in some detail in the chapter, firstly by outlining Freud's own argument and then looking at how it has been taken up by other analysts, especially in the French tradition. More specifically, I discuss how Laplanche has used it to support his more general theory of childhood seduction, which is essentially a return to Freud's 'original' theory of trauma. And although Lacan has often been credited with restoring the idea of *Nachträglichkeit* as a central concept in psychoanalysis, my argument in this chapter is that this is not so much in relation to trauma but, rather, in relation to the operation of language, desire and the drive.

The question of *causality* is especially problematic in relation to *Nachträglichkeit* because some authors have argued that it involves a process of 'reverse causality', which is something I discuss in the chapter along with the question regarding the status of an 'original trauma'. I conclude by examining the relationship of *Nachträglichkeit* and trauma to history. I briefly discuss Miller's concept of history as 'hystory'; Caruth's idea of history as a way to fill the void of the trauma, with a particular reference to her reading of Freud's *Moses and Monotheism*; and Lawrence Langer's idea of chronological and durational time in relation to the experience of the Holocaust.

Chapter 7 concludes this work and here I argue that the traumatic neuroses represent an irruption of the Real into the Symbolic-Imaginary order. Unlike many instances of psychosis, such an irruption tends to be transitory but, even so, deeply unsettling and troubling for the subject. And this irruption of the Real into the Symbolic-Imaginary is brought about through the operation of the drive in its incessant 'scraping' of surplus jouissance from the Symbolic-Imaginary universe (the 'external world'). The traumatic effects of this irruption are due to failure of language to fully decipher such jouissance.

Although it could be (and has been) argued that the traumatic neuroses are simply a Freudian 'version' of PTSD, my argument is that the difference lies in the fact that the theory of the traumatic neuroses provides a way to show how the drive and the 'external world' are intricately linked to one another, whereas the 'PTSD paradigm', as I call it, maintains a clear demarcation between the 'external' and the 'internal'. And although this is primarily a *theoretical* rather than a *clinical* work (and is certainly not a 'manual' on how to 'treat' trauma), in the concluding section I do briefly touch upon the question of whether a traumatic neurosis should be seen as a clinical structure in its own right.

2

The Traumatic Neuroses

Introduction

As I noted in the Introduction there is a broad and complex Freudian legacy with regards to trauma, including, ironically perhaps, within PTSD itself. There are a range of 'psychoanalytically inspired' (for want of a better term) therapies which draw to varying degrees upon Freud's work on trauma, although one of the difficulties all such approaches share, I would argue, is dealing with the question of Freud's (alleged) abandonment of his 'childhood seduction theory' in 1897. I will have more to say about this question shortly, but for now I would just like to state that one of my key arguments in this chapter (and in the book as a whole) is that Freud's theory of the traumatic neuroses, especially as it developed in his later work, is clear evidence he never completely 'abandoned' his theory of childhood seduction as the origins of adult psychopathology; rather, the evolution of his theory of the psychoneuroses demonstrates his growing recognition of the key importance of psychical processes (repression, the unconscious, the operation of the drives, and so on) in the (re)construction of the subject's history.

© The Author(s), under exclusive license to Springer Nature Switzerland AG 2025

L. Chapman, *Traumatic Neurosis Revisited*, The Palgrave Lacan Series,
https://doi.org/10.1007/978-3-031-89158-8_2

On the other hand, I think it is fair to argue that Freud's use of the terms 'traumatic neuroses' and 'traumatic neurosis' in his later work signal a change in *emphasis* (if not *substance*) in the way he viewed trauma and this is something I will be discussing at the end of this chapter. I will begin my discussion, however, by briefly reviewing Freud's earlier work on trauma before exploring his use of the term 'traumatic neurosis', both 'pre' and 'post' *Beyond the Pleasure Principle*, which seems to mark a significant shift in his use of the term. I then discuss a particular example of the traumatic neuroses, the so-called 'war neuroses', which Freud and his colleagues hoped they could use to refute a commonly held view (propagated by psychoanalysis' growing number of opponents) that the war neuroses disproved a key element of Freud's theory, namely that the aetiology of the psychoneuroses were rooted in childhood sexual conflicts. I then turn to the rather more problematic concept of the actual neuroses their relation to the traumatic neuroses, with a particular focus on Verhaeghe and Vanheule's argument regarding actual neurosis and PTSD.

Situating Trauma in Freud's Work

Freud adopted the terms 'trauma' and 'traumatic', as in referring to psychical 'wounds', early on in his work. For example, in his draft letter to Fliess *The Neuroses of Defence*, in the course of a more general discussion about the role of repression in neuroses he writes, "The course taken by the illness in neuroses of repression is in general always the same: (1) the sexual experience (or series of experiences), which is traumatic and premature and is to be repressed…"[1] And in his *Project for a Scientific Psychology* the term trauma appears several times in his discussion of the 'Emma' case:

> Now, this case is typical of repression in hysteria. We invariably find that a memory is repressed which has only become a trauma by *deferred action*.[2]

[1] Sigmund Freud, *The Complete Letters of Sigmund Freud to Wilhelm Fliess 1887–1904*, trans. Jeffrey M. Masson (Cambridge, Massachusetts: The Belkap Press of Harvard University Press, 1985), 164.

[2] I will return to the question of 'deferred action' a bit later in this text when I briefly discuss Freud's concept of *Nachträglichkeit* and as one of my concluding questions.

> The cause of this state of things is the retardation of puberty as compared with the rest of the individual's development.[3]

And further on:

> Now analysis indicates that what is disturbing in a sexual trauma is evidently the release of affect; and experience teaches us to recognize hysterics as individuals of whom one knows in part that they have become *prematurely* sexually excitable owing to mechanical and emotional stimulation (masturbation), and of whom one can assume in part that a premature sexual release is present in their innate disposition.[4]

In their 'Preliminary Communication' which introduces *Studies on Hysteria*, Freud and Breuer argue that the aetiology of hysteria is to be found at least partially in psychical traumas.[5] Furthermore, at this early stage of his work Freud emphasises, along with Breuer, the *accidental* and *external* nature of the origins of such traumas. For example, when discussing what they have learnt from working with hypnotised hysterical patients they write:

> They (the case studies with hysterical patients) are valuable theoretically because they have taught us that external events determine the pathology of hysteria to an extent far greater than is known and recognized. It is of course obvious that in cases of 'traumatic' hysteria what provokes the symptoms is the accident. The causal connection is equally evident in hysterical attacks when it is possible to gather from the patient's utterances that in each attack he is hallucinating the same event which provoked the first one. The situation is more obscure in the case of other phenomena.[6]

They argue that it is not necessarily just one major traumatic event that may provoke a hysteria; instead, it can be a number of 'partial' traumas. They also point out that:

---

[3] Sigmund Freud, 'Project for a Scientific Psychology', in *The Standard Edition of the Complete Psychological Works of Sigmund Freud* (London: Hogarth Press, 1950), I, 356, italics in original.

[4] *Ibid.*, 357, italics in original.

[5] Sigmund Freud and Josef Breuer, "Studies on Hysteria," in *The Standard Edition of the Complete Psychological Works of Sigmund Freud*, vol. II (London: Hogarth Press, 1895).

[6] *Ibid.*, 3–4.

> ...the causal relation between the determining psychical trauma and the hysterical phenomenon is not of a kind implying that the trauma merely acts like an *agent provocateur* in releasing the symptom, which thereafter leads an independent existence. We must presume rather that the psychical trauma—or more precisely the memory of the trauma—acts like a foreign body which long after its entry must continue to be regarded as an agent that is still at work...[7]

As Laplanche and Pontalis point out, up until Freud's (in)famous 'abandonment' of his 'seduction theory' in 1897 he believed that many of his patients' neuroses were rooted in childhood sexual experiences. Furthermore, these experiences, because of the age of the child, are experienced *passively*:

> That the scene of seduction is experienced passively means not only that the subject behaves in a passive way during it, but also that he undergoes it without its being able to evoke a response in him, since no corresponding sexual ideas are available: the state of passivity implies an absence of preparation, and the seduction produces 'sexual fright' (*Sexualschreck*).
>
> Such is the importance attached by Freud to (childhood) seduction in the genesis of repression that he looks systematically for scenes of passive seduction in obsessional neurosis as well as in hysteria, where they first came to light.[8]

For example, in his draft letter to Fliess, which I cited earlier, Freud argues, in relation to repression in obsessional neurosis:

> The repression may come about owing to the memory of the pleasure itself releasing unpleasure when it is reproduced in later years; this should be explicable by a theory of sexuality. But things may happen differently as well. In *all* my cases of obsessional neurosis, at a very early age, years before the experience of pleasure, there had been *purely passive* experience; and this can hardly be accidental.[9]

---

[7] *Ibid.*, 6.

[8] Laplanche and Pontalis, *The Language of Psychoanalysis*, 405.

[9] Freud, *The Complete Letters*, 165, italics in original.

In other words, Freud is arguing that even though psychical 'working over',[10] that is, the work of repression, fantasy and retranscription[11] plays an important role in the construction of a neurosis, at root there is an actual sexual experience.

According to psychoanalytic folklore, all this was to change on 21 September 1897 when Freud wrote in a letter to Fliess:

> And now I want to confide in you immediately the great secret that has been slowly dawning upon me in the last few months. I no longer believe in my *neurotica* [Freud's theory of the neuroses]. This is probably not intelligible without an explanation: after all, you yourself found credible what I was able to tell you.[12]

Freud's explanation hinged on several different factors: firstly, he refers to his 'continual disappointments' in bringing his analyses with his patients to a 'real conclusion' (although he doesn't explain why this necessarily meant his *neurotica* was wrong); secondly, he simply couldn't bring himself to believe that all his patients' fathers must have been 'perverts' (paedophiles, sexual abusers) in order to account for the frequency of the hysteria he was encountering; thirdly "…the certain insight that there are no indications of reality in the unconscious, so that one cannot distinguish between truth and fiction that has been cathected with affect."[13] This introduced the idea that unconscious fantasy had a large role to play in his patients' 'recollection' of childhood trauma. And fourthly:

> …in the most deep-going psychosis the unconscious memory does not break through, so that the secret of childhood experiences is not disclosed even in the most confused delirium. If one thus sees that the unconscious never overcomes the resistance of the conscious, the expectation that in

[10] Here I am following Laplanche and Pontalis' argument in *The Language of Psychoanalysis* that, "Understood very broadly, psychical working out (or over) might be said to cover all of the operations of the psychical apparatus." (366). However, they are also clear that Freud's specific use of the term was in reference to the transformation of energy through binding or diversion.

[11] The process of *Nachträglichkeit* which I will return to shortly.

[12] Freud, *The Complete Letters*, 264.

[13] *Ibid.*, 264.

> treatment the opposite is bound to happen, to the point where the unconscious is completely tamed by the conscious, also diminishes.[14]

This letter has been seized upon by many of Freud's outspoken critics and added fuel to the flames of the 'Freud wars' which underwent a resurgence in the 1980s.[15] For many feminists and survivors of child sexual abuse in particular, Freud's apparent rejection of the reality of childhood sexual trauma was evidence that psychoanalysis itself was no longer helpful in tackling the problem of such abuse. As Laplanche and Pontalis argue in their discussion of Freud's childhood seduction theory that I cited earlier:

> It is traditional to look upon Freud's dropping of the seduction theory in 1897 as a decisive step in the foundation of psycho-analytic theory, and in the bringing to the fore of such conceptions as unconscious phantasy, psychical reality, spontaneous infantile sexuality and so on. Freud himself asserted the importance of this moment in the history of his thought on several occasions: 'If hysterical subjects trace back their symptoms to traumas that are fictitious, then the new factg which emerges is precisely that they create such scenes in phantasy, and this psychical reality requires to be taken into account alongside practical reality.[16]

And Freud's remarks on this subject in the opening part of his *On the History of the Psycho-Analytic Movement* seem to confirm his abandonment of the theory:

> If hysterical subjects trace back their symptoms to traumas that are fictitious, then the new fact which emerges is precisely that they create such scenes in *phantasy*, and this psychical reality requires to be taken into account alongside practical reality. This reflection was soon followed by the discovery that these phantasies were intended to cover up the auto-erotic

---

[14] *Ibid.*, 265.

[15] See for example Jeffrey Masson's vitriolic attack on Freud's so-called abandonment of the seduction theory: Jeffrey M. Masson, *The Assault on Truth: Freud's Suppression of the Seduction Theory* (New York: Farrar, Strauss & Giroux, 1984).

[16] Laplanche and Pontalis, *The Language of Psychoanalysis*, 405–406.

activity of the first years of childhood, to embellish it and raise it to a higher plane. And now, from behind the phantasies, the whole range of a child's sexual life came to light'.[17]

However, as Karin Ahbel-Rappe points out in her paper on Freud's seduction theory, the question of whether or not he really did 'abandon' his belief that his patients' neuroses were rooted in actual childhood sexual experiences is a contested one. She argues that:

> Recent accounts of the seduction theory and the question of its abandonment have emphasized the continuity of Freud's work before and after the seduction theory, claiming that Freud did not abandon his concern with the event of seduction but rather came to appreciate that an understanding of fantasy was *also* essential.[18]

Although Ahbel-Rappe disagrees with such 'continuist' arguments, and argues instead that Freud "...theoretically nullified the value of the difference between real and fantasised seduction",[19] in my view she fails to make a convincing case that Freud had actually 'abandoned' his initial theory. Arguing, for example, that "...Freud, for the most part, did abandon the passionate concerns of his early theorizing on seduction"[20] simply raises more questions than it answers. Just because Freud may have become less 'passionate' about his theory of childhood seduction does not mean he no longer believed such 'seductions' were not an important factor in the emergence of neuroses.

And Laplanche and Pontalis note: "Right up to the end of his life, Freud continued to assert the existence, prevalence and pathogenic force of scenes of seduction actually experienced by children." And, furthermore"... Freud could never resign himself to treating phantasy as the

[17] Sigmund Freud, "On the History of the Psychoanalytic Movement," in *The Standard Edition of the Complete Psychological Works of Sigmund Freud*, vol. XIV (London: Hogarth Press, 1914), 3–66.

[18] Karin Ahbel-Rappe, '"I No Longer Believe": Did Freud Abandon the Seduction Theory?', *Journal of the American Psychoanalytic Association*, 54.1 (2006), 171–199, italics in original.

[19] *Ibid.*, 171

[20] *Ibid.*, 192.

pure and simple outgrowth of the spontaneous sexual life of the child. He is forever searching, behind the phantasy, for whatever has founded it in its reality...."[21]

They then go on to argue that:

> ...the crucial question is to decide whether the seduction-phantasy has to be considered merely as a defensive and projective distortion of the positive component of the Oedipus complex or whether it is to be treated as the transposed expression of a fundamental datum, namely, the fact that the child's sexuality is entirely organised by something which comes to it, as it were, *from the outside*: the relationship between the parents, and the parents' wishes which pre-date and determine the form of the wishes of the subject. Viewed from this angle, seductions really experienced as well as seduction-phantasies become nothing more than concrete expressions of this basic fact.[22]

In other words, at least according to my reading, it is not a case of an 'either/or'; that is, *either* there is an actual event in the subject's early childhood, *or* such an event is constructed in phantasy at a later date. Rather, the 'childhood trauma' is probably best viewed as complex interweaving of phantasy and actuality; something *did* happen, but not necessarily in the manner that it is recalled later-on by the subject. And this idea of both phantasy and actuality being constitutive in the aetiology of trauma is suggested by Freud in his *Introductory Lectures,* which occurred well after his apparent 'abandonment' of the childhood seduction theory and prior to the re-emergence of trauma as a key concept in *Beyond the Pleasure Principle*. For example, in lecture 18 he discusses the role that (actual) trauma may have in the formation of neurosis but then goes onto question whether it is that simple by using the example of a girl with a fixation on her father:

> On the one hand, a little girl's being in love like this with her father is something so common and so frequently surmounted that the term 'traumatic' applied to it would lose all its meaning; and on the other hand,

---

[21] Laplanche and Pontalis, *The Language of Psychoanalysis*, 406–407.

[22] *Ibid.,* 407, my italics.

> the patient's history showed us that in the first instance her erotic fixation appeared to have passed off without doing any damage, and it was only several years later that it reappeared in the symptoms of the obsessional neurosis. Here, then, we foresee complications, a greater wealth of determinants for the onset of illness; but we may also suspect that there is no need to abandon the traumatic line of approach as being erroneous: it must be possible to fit it in and subsume it somewhere else.[23]

There is, however, another important reason to question Freud's so-called 'abandonment' of the idea of actual childhood trauma, and this is the fact that he was questioning the 'actuality' of such experiences from very early on in his work. And much of this questioning revolves around the concept of *Nachträglichkeit* (erroneously translated as 'deferred action' in Strachey's translation), which makes its first appearance in the *Project* in 1895 and his account of the 'Emma' case which I referred to earlier. I shall be exploring the concept of *Nachträglichkeit* in some detail further on in this work, but very briefly it is the idea that a psychical trauma is constructed *retroactively*; the original event, for example a childhood sexual experience, may well have occurred but it is not registered by the subject at the time as 'traumatic'. It is only at a later date, which according to Freud is post-puberty, when another event occurs that has some association with the original one, that a 'temporal looping back' occurs, in the form of a chain of signifiers, from the second event to the first, which constructs a 'traumatic' memory of the first event. And it is this (retroactively constructed) memory that traumatises the subject in the here-and-now. *Nachträglichkeit* is important for two reasons: firstly, it shows clearly that Freud never subscribed to a 'naïve' theory of trauma, that is, the idea that psychical trauma, and any associated psychopathology, is purely the result of an 'objective', physical event that occurred at some point in the subject's past. Secondly, and leading on from this, it shows that trauma is the result of a complex process, which has both 'objective' and 'subjective' aspects.

---

[23] Sigmund Freud, "Introductory Lectures on Psycho-Analysis," in *The Standard Edition of the Complete Psychological Works of Sigmund Freud*, vol. XVI (London: Hogarth Press, 1916–1917).

Freud's Theory of the Traumatic Neuroses

Having discussed Freud's initial approach to trauma and the question of whether or not he 'abandoned' the idea that the roots of trauma lay in actual, childhood events, I would now like to turn to his idea of the traumatic neuroses. In many ways this seems to further challenge the idea that he 'abandoned' his original theory of childhood trauma, but on the other hand it seems to complicate things because the emphasis shifts to the 'traumatic events' themselves, or, as I prefer to call them, the 'wounds of life'. Furthermore, the focus is no longer on early childhood experiences but rather on experiences in the here-and-now, or at least post-puberty.

Laplanche and Pontalis note in their entry on the subject in *The Language of Psychoanalysis* that the term 'traumatic neurosis' predates psychoanalysis and has been used in psychiatry to refer to events that make incursions upon the subject's psychical organisation.[24] They point out that here the term 'traumatic' is being used metaphorically, because the medical concept of trauma refers to *physical* wounding, which in neuropsychiatry would include traumas to the central nervous system. With regards to traumatic neurosis in the psychical sense, they argue that one of the key issues is what they call the 'trauma-disposition problem', by which they mean the extent to which an external event can 'trigger' an underlying psychopathology. They link this to the more fundamental difficulty in trying to differentiate between the *traumatic* and *actual* neuroses, which is something I will be returning to later in this chapter. They also question the need for the term at all because psychoanalysis "…contests the decisive function of the traumatic event."[25] This is because the effect of the traumatic event seems to be related to the subject's tolerance of it, and, furthermore, the traumatic experience has to be situated within the subject's particular psychical organisation and history. They then go onto to discuss the appearances of the term in Freud's writings and at this

[24] Jean Laplanche and Jean-Bertrand Pontalis, *The Language of Psychoanalysis* (London: Karnac Books, 1988), 470–473.

[25] *Ibid.*, 472.

point I think it would be helpful to look at some of these in order to get a sense of how the idea has developed.

It is important to note that prior to his 'abandonment' of his theory of childhood seduction in 1897, which I discussed earlier, Freud was using the terms 'traumatic neuroses' and 'traumatic neurosis' almost interchangeably with 'psychoneuroses', that is, hysteria and obsessional neurosis. It is only after this turning point that the terms appear to take on a different meaning.

In Freud's pre-psychoanalytic writings he makes a brief reference to Hofrat Meynert's paper on traumatic neurosis during his review of August Forel's theory of hypnotism.[26] He also makes a reference to the entry 'Neurosis, traumatic' in Burn's *Lexikon* in the context of his (Freud's) paper on hypnosis.[27] In his Letter 18 to Fliess Freud introduces a new concept, 'conflagration' (which according to Strachey is the only reference to the term in the Standard Edition) as one of the four 'general aspects' of the neuroses:

> ...it means conditions of what might be called acute degeneration (for example, in severe intoxication, in fevers, in the prestages of paralysis)—catastrophes, that is, in which there occur disturbances of the sexual affects without sexual precipitating causes. *Traumatic neurosis might possibly be approached from this point of view.*[28]

However, it is only in *Studies on Hysteria* that the terms 'traumatic neurosis' and 'traumatic neuroses' really comes to the fore. In their 'Preliminary Communication' Freud and Breuer argue that external events "determine the pathology of hysteria to an extent far greater than is known and recognized."[29] Here the reference is to 'traumatic hysteria' but further down Freud does use the term 'traumatic neuroses'. The gist of Freud and Breuer's argument is that that the hysterical symptoms presented by their

[26] Sigmund Freud, "Review of August Forel's Hypnotism," in *The Standard Edition of the Complete Psychological Works of Sigmund Freud*, vol. I (London: Hogarth Press, 1889), 91–102.

[27] Sigmund Freud, "Hypnosis," in *The Standard Edition of the Complete Psychological Works of Sigmund Freud*, vol. I (London: Hogarth Press, 1889), 104–14.

[28] Freud, *The Complete Letters*, 75, my italics.

[29] Freud and Breuer, 'Studies on Hysteria', 4.

patients are the product of an earlier, external trauma, and they make reference to a number of case studies that make up the main body of *Studies on Hysteria.*

> *Our experiences have shown us, however, that the most various symptoms, which are ostensibly spontaneous and, as one might say, idiopathic products of hysteria, are just as strictly related to the precipitating trauma as the phenomena to which we have just alluded and which exhibit the connection quite clearly.*[30]

It is clear that at this stage of Freud's thinking, he views trauma as something 'external', that is, related to one or more events in the world. In this sense the term 'traumatic' seems somewhat superfluous because at this stage of Freud's thinking *all* psychoneuroses would appear to have their origins in some form of external event. This is something I will return to later on when I discuss the need for such a term in the first place.

Freud and Breuer go onto argue that in some cases the precipitating cause (of the psychoneurosis) is not so obvious and instead there is what they describe as a 'symbolic relation' between the cause and the presenting symptoms. They give the examples of neuralgia following mental pain and vomiting following feelings of moral disgust. And in yet other cases the precipitating cause is far from clear:

> It is precisely the typical hysterical symptoms which fall into this class, such as hemi-anaesthesia, contraction of the field of vision, epileptiform convulsions, and so on. An explanation of our views on this group must be reserved for a fuller discussion of the subject.[31]

Further on in the text Freud and Breuer make reference to traumatic neurosis in the context of *psychically acquired hysteria*:

> We have found, however, that a severe trauma (such as occurs in a traumatic neurosis) or a laborious suppression (as of a sexual affect, for instance)

[30] *Ibid.*, 4, italics in original.

[31] *Ibid.*, 5

> can bring about a splitting-off of groups of ideas even in people who are in other respects unaffected; and this would be the mechanism of *psychically acquired* hysteria.[32]

In the first of the case histories (Fräulein Anna O) Breuer makes reference to Charcot's theory of traumatic hysteria in context of paralysis of the patient's arm. In the theoretical part of the text, in the section on hysterical conversion he makes reference to hysterical symptoms of traumatic origin: "The term 'traumatic hysteria' has already been applied to phenomena, which, as being consequences of physical injuries—traumas in the narrowest sense of the word—form part of the class of 'traumatic neuroses'".[33]

Finally, in the section on unconscious ideas Breuer makes reference to the Anna O case and argues that it throws light on traumatic neurosis:

> During the first few days after the traumatic event, the state of hypnoid fright is repeated every time the event is recalled. While this state recurs more and more often, its intensity so far diminishes that it no longer *alternates* with waking thought but only exists side by side with it. It now becomes continuous, and the somatic symptoms, which earlier were only present during the attack of fright, acquire a permanent existence.[34]

It is important to note here that Breuer is referring to 'the traumatic *event*'. This is a good example of the more fundamental position that Freud and Breuer held towards trauma at this time in Freud's teaching; that is, that the event has a causal role in the production of trauma. Furthermore, such events are 'external' insofar as they are occurring in the 'world' and impacting upon the subject. Clearly, terms such as 'external' and 'world' are themselves problematic, which is why Lacan sought to find various ways to circumvent them, for example, with his concept of *extimacy* and the use of models such as the torus and the Moebius strip—something I will discuss in more detail in the Conclusion.

---

[32] *Ibid.,* 12–13, italics in original.

[33] *Ibid.,* 209.

[34] *Ibid.,* 235, italics in original.

In lecture 18 of his *Introductory Lectures* Freud discusses the idea of a 'fixation' to a trauma and drawing on the case of the Anna O case to illustrate his point. He argues that this kind of 'fixation' can also be found in cases of traumatic neurosis, and cites both the ongoing Great War and pre-war accidents as examples:

> Traumatic neuroses are not in their essence the same thing as the spontaneous neuroses which we are in the habit of investigating and treating by analysis…But in one respect we may insist that there is a complete agreement between them. The traumatic neuroses give a clear indication that a fixation to the moment of the traumatic accident lies at their root. These patients regularly repeat the traumatic situation in their dreams; where hysteriform occur that admit of an analysis, we find that the attack corresponds to a complete transplanting of the patient into the traumatic situation.[35]

It is not altogether clear what Freud is getting at here. On the one hand he seems to be suggesting that the traumatic neuroses are different from the psychoneuroses (although for some reason he uses the term 'spontaneous neuroses' instead), whereas on the other hand he states that a 'fixation' on the traumatic event can occur in both cases, something that is clearly demonstrated in his *Studies on Hysteria* case examples. In the same lecture Freud also notes that although in some cases the neurosis could be directly related to the traumatic event, in other cases things are more complicated because, for example, there can be a time gap between the 'original' trauma (and the 'original' fixation) and the development of pathological symptoms. Although not made explicit, this appears to be a reference to his idea of *Nachträglichkeit*, which I will be exploring in a later chapter. However, Freud goes on to argue that in spite of such complications "…we may also suspect that there is no need to abandon the traumatic line of approach as being erroneous: it must be possible to fit it in and subsume it somewhere else."[36] In other words, Freud seems to be making it clear, nearly twenty years after his so-called 'abandonment' of

[35] Freud, 'Introductory Lectures', 274–275.

[36] *Ibid.*, 276.

his childhood seduction theory, that real events in the subject's history place a role in the aetiology of trauma.

In lecture 24 Freud discusses the relationship between the ego and neuroses, and argues that in the case of the traumatic neuroses "...we are unmistakably presented with a self-interested motive on the part of the ego, seeking for protection and advantage..."[37] He goes on to argue that although such a self-interested motive cannot create the neurosis by itself it can 'assent' to it and 'maintain' it. The motive in question is to protect the ego from the traumatic situation that precipitated the neurosis in the first place and "...it will not allow recovery to occur until a repetition of these dangers seems no longer possible or until compensation has been received for the danger that has been endured."[38]

The reference to 'compensation' is especially interesting in this context. It is not clear whether Freud was referring to financial compensation, but he could well have been because one of his original examples of a traumatic event were railway accidents, which had already featured in a long-running controversy regarding the aetiology of so-called 'railway spine' in the latter part of the nineteenth century and that had related closely to the question of financial compensation from the railway companies.[39]

In his *Three Essays* Freud discusses the sources of excitation that can contribute to infantile sexuality and argues that mechanical excitation, for example, riding in carriages (horse drawn or railway) can give rise of a pleasurable sensation that is clearly sexual. However, he then goes onto to add that a combination of fright and mechanical agitation can produce a traumatic neurosis: "It may be at least assumed that these influences, which, when they are of small intensity, become sources of sexual excitation, lead to a profound disorder in the sexual mechanism or chemistry if they operate with exaggerated force."[40]

---

[37] *Ibid.*, 382.

[38] *Ibid.*, 382.

[39] See for example Thomas Keller's paper on 'railway spine' in the United States in the nineteenth century which focuses on the arguments over whether it was a physical or psychological illness, and how this related to the question of compensation from the railway companies. Keller, Thomas, 'Railway Spine Revisited: Traumatic Neurosis or Neurotrauma?', *Journal of the History of Medicine and Allied Sciences*, 50.4 (1995), 507–524.

[40] Sigmund Freud, 'Three Essays on the Theory of Sexuality', in *The Standard Edition of the Complete Psychological Works of Sigmund Freud* (London: Hogarth Press, 1905), VII, 202.

Here, Freud shows that there is a relationship between sexual excitation and trauma; or, more to the point, that when sexual excitation goes beyond a certain limit it becomes traumatic, overwhelming—which is essentially his argument in *Beyond the Pleasure Principle.* This line of argument also opens up the possibility that 'external' excitations, in this case riding in a carriage, can be linked to 'internal' ones, that is, the drive. This is something I will return to shortly in my discussion of the war neuroses.

Early on in *Beyond the Pleasure Principle* Freud makes reference to the traumatic neuroses in the context of severe concussions, railway accidents and other life-threating situations. He also makes reference to the Great War which had just ended and which gave rise to numerous incidences of traumatic neurosis. He remarks that such neuroses "…at least put an end to the temptation to attribute the cause of the disorder to organic lesions of the nervous system brought about by mechanical force."[41]

He goes on to argue that the traumatic neuroses are characterised by fright or 'surprise' as the key causative factor. He also comments on the fact that the dreams in traumatic neurosis take the subject back to the traumatic situation, which is somewhat puzzling if the function of dreams is wish-fulfilment:

> If we are not to be shaken in our belief in the wish-fulfilling tenor of dreams by the dreams of traumatic neurotics, we still have one resource open to us: we may argue that the function of dreaming, like so much else, is upset in this condition and diverted from its purpose, or we may be driven to reflect on the mysterious masochistic trends of the ego.[42]

In other words, Freud is arguing that trauma essentially 'disables' this function of dreams (wish fulfilment), which is very close to his argument that (external) trauma disrupts or disables the pleasure principle. At the same time, though, he is at pains to point out that traumatic neurosis does not equate with what he describes as the 'old, naive theory of shock',

[41] Sigmund Freud, 'Beyond the Pleasure Principle', in *The Standard Edition of the Complete Psychological Works of Sigmund Freud* (London: Hogarth Press, 1920), XVIII, 12.

[42] *Ibid.*, 13–14.

whereby the trauma remains at the physical level in the form of, for example, direct damage to the molecular structure of nervous system. Rather, for Freud the trauma is at the psychical level and "…is caused by lack of any preparedness for anxiety, including lack of hypercathexis of the systems that would be the first to receive the stimulus."[43]

In other words, the trauma is linked to the *unpreparedness* of the subject (how Freud defines fright), not the 'physicality' of the traumatic event itself. This is why Freud argues that anxiety is a protection against trauma, because it helps prepare the subject for the event. Freud also argues that any physical wound or injury inflicted at the time of the 'traumatic'event tends to mitigate the development of psychical trauma (in the form of a neurosis). In other words, those individuals suffering from *physical* trauma are less likely to suffer from *psychical* trauma. Freud's argument is that:

> …on the one hand, the mechanical violence of the trauma would liberate a quantity of sexual excitation which, owing to the lack of preparation for anxiety, would have a traumatic effect; but, on the other hand, the simultaneous physical injury, by calling for a narcissistic hypercathexis of the injured organ, would bind the excess of excitation.[44]

In other words, the 'narcissistic hypercathexis' of the physical injury and its binding function 'counteracts' the unbinding effect of the release of sexual excitation produced by the traumatic event.

In their paper on the paradigm shift in the conceptualisation of trauma in the twentieth century, Edgar Jones and Simon Wessely argue that follow-up research suggests that Freud was wrong to argue that physical injury can counteract the psychical one: "Although soldiers recovering from wounds appeared to be free of neurosis, once an injury had healed, psychological disorders often emerged."[45] However, this seems to be based on a misreading of Freud's argument as articulated in the quote

[43] *Ibid.*, 31.

[44] *Ibid.*, 33.

[45] Edgar Jones and Simon Wessely, 'A Paradigm Shift in the Conceptualization of Psychological Trauma in the twentieth Century', *Journal of Anxiety Disorders*, 21.2 (2007), 164–75, p.168.

above; in fact, in some ways it would appear to *vindicate* it, insofar that once the injured physical organ has healed there is no longer a need for the 'narcissistic hypercathexis' that binds the excitation. In other words, the traumatic (sexual) excitation caused by the original 'mechanical agitation', that is, the external event, is counteracted by the hypercathexis of the affected physical organ, but once the injury has healed the sexual energy (which in Freudian parlance is the libido) becomes unbound and thus traumatises the subject.

In *Beyond the Pleasure Principle* Freud argues that (psychical) trauma is a 'breach' of the shield which protects the 'living vesicle' (which appears to equate with the cortical layer, and which, according to Freud, is later to become the system *Cs*) from external stimuli or excitations. However, there are also excitations coming from *within* the psychical apparatus (for want of a better word) from which there is no such protection. It is only in *Inhibitions, Symptoms and Anxiety*, that Freud will provide some clarity regarding the relationship between 'external' and 'internal' sources of trauma.

At this point it is worth quoting in full what is probably Freud's most definitive definition of trauma:

> We describe as 'traumatic' any excitations from outside which are powerful enough to break through the protective shield. It seems to me that the concept of trauma necessarily implies a connection of this kind with a breach in an otherwise efficacious barrier against stimuli. Such an event as an external trauma is bound to provoke a disturbance on a large scale in the functioning of the organism's energy and to set in motion every possible defensive measure. At the same time, the pleasure principle is for the moment put out of action.[46]

However, at this point in Freud's argument it is still not clear whether a *traumatic* neurosis would also be considered a *psychoneurosis*. There is no indication thus far in Freud's argument that an external 'shock' or 'excitation' is subjected to repression or any other form of psychical 'working over'. Rather, it would appear that such a shock/excitation directly

---

[46] Freud, 'Beyond the Pleasure Principle', 29.

'traumatises' the subject (or, as Freud would be more likely to put it, the psychical apparatus), in the here-and-now.

In *Inhibitions, Symptoms and Anxiety*, written in 1925 and first published in February 1926, Freud essentially consolidates his arguments regarding trauma. As I indicated earlier, in *Beyond the Pleasure Principle* Freud *does* argue that there are excitations coming from 'within'. However, in that text Freud is still using the term 'traumatic' to refer to *external* excitations (stimuli) and, for some reason, does not apply this term to the *internal* excitations, even though he acknowledges their existence. In fact, he does not even refer to such excitations as emanating from the drives. In contrast, in *Inhibitions, Symptoms and Anxiety* the term 'traumatic' refers to *both* external *and* internal stimuli, although the ego's response to each type of stimuli is radically different. Freud's argument is complex and evolves over the course of the whole paper and in fact it is only in the text's Addenda that he finally consolidates his theory. Here he argues that trauma is linked to a sense of *helplessness* in the subject in the face of a danger; *physical* helplessness if the danger is 'real', by which Freud means 'external', and *psychical* helplessness if the danger is 'instinctual', that is, emanating from the drives. However, Freud also argues that these two types of danger can be linked or 'mingled' with one another. In these situations:

> The danger is known and real but the anxiety in regard to it is over-great, greater than seems proper to us. It is this surplus of anxiety which betrays the presence of a neurotic element. Such cases, however, introduce no new principle; for analysis shows that to the known real danger an unknown instinctual one is attached.[47]

The last sentence of this quote is particularly interesting because it echoes something Freud discusses earlier on in his paper and suggests that there may be a relationship between 'external' and 'internal' traumas. In part VII of his paper Freud briefly discusses the question of the war (traumatic) neuroses in the context of anxiety as a reaction of the ego to

[47] Sigmund Freud, 'Inhibitions, Symptoms and Anxiety', in *The Standard Edition of the Complete Psychological Works of Sigmund Freud* (London: Hogarth Press, 1926), XX, 165–166.

danger and acknowledges that for many commentators (some of whom were already opposed to psychoanalysis) the traumas of war and the immediate threat to life had 'disapproved' the idea of a sexual aetiology for the neuroses. However, he goes onto to argue that "…it would seem highly improbable that a neurosis could come into being merely because of the objective presence of danger, without any participation of the deeper levels of the mental apparatus."[48]

As with his later remarks in the Addenda regarding the 'intermingling' of the two sources of trauma (physical and psychical), Freud is tantalisingly elusive by what exactly he is referring to in the phrase "participation of the deeper levels of the mental apparatus". In my view this suggests that Freud is still struggling, some thirty years later, with the problem of 'real' trauma, in spite of his so-called abandonment of his 'seduction theory' in 1897. In other words, perhaps Freud is still trying to work out exactly how such 'real', that is, external, events (for example, childhood sexual abuse) are linked to internal psychical mechanisms.

Freud continued to make references to the traumatic neuroses up until the end of his life, the last one being in *An Outline of Psychoanalysis*, where he argues that the traumatic neuroses may be the exception to the rule that every neurosis has its roots in childhood experiences, though he also points out that there is not enough evidence to prove this either way.[49] In lecture 29 of *New Introductory Lectures* Freud makes reference to traumatic neurosis in the context of dreams. He reiterates his argument that the dreams in traumatic neurosis are the only genuine exception to the rule of dreams being wish fulfilments. However, he goes onto argue that this is because the wish fulfilment function of dream *fails* in these particular cases:

> We say that a dream is the fulfilment of a wish; but if you want to take these latter objections (that some dreams are not wish fulfilments) into account, you can say nevertheless that a dream is an *attempt* at the fulfil-

---

[48] *Ibid.*, 129.

[49] Sigmund Freud, "An Outline of Psycho-Analysis," in *The Standard Edition of the Complete Psychological Works of Sigmund Freud*, vol. XXII (London: Hogarth Press, 1940), 141–207.

> ment of a wish ... In certain circumstances a dream is only able to put its intention into effect very incompletely, or must abandon it entirely...In these circumstances it will happen that one cannot sleep, that one gives up sleep from dread of the failure of the function of dreaming. Traumatic neuroses are here offering us an extreme case; but we must admit that childhood experiences, too, are of a traumatic nature...[50]

In *Moses and Monotheism* Freud makes reference to traumatic neurosis in the context of 'delayed trauma', which is also related to *Nachträglichkeit* (though Freud does not use the term here):

> ...in spite of the fundamental differences between the two cases—the problem of traumatic neurosis and that of Jewish monotheism—there is nevertheless one point of agreement: namely, in the characteristic that might be described as 'latency'. According to our assured hypothesis, in the history of the Jewish religion there was a long period after the defection from the religion of Moses during which no sign was to be detected of the monotheist idea...[51]

It is important to note that here Freud is not arguing that Jewish monotheism is the product of a traumatic neurosis (resulting from, according to Freud, the murder of Moses) but, rather, that they are both characterised by 'latency' (which seems to be another way to describe *Nachträglichkeit*).

So, it is clear that Freud retained the idea of traumatic neurosis throughout his life. And in doing so, I would argue, he retained the connection between 'external' events and 'internal' trauma. However, one of the problems with maintaining this connection is that the concept of the *traumatic* neuroses can easily be conflated with that of the *actual* neuroses, which in Freud's view were outside the remit of psychoanalytic treatment. Before exploring this in more detail however, I would like to spend

---

[50] Sigmund Freud, 'New Introductory Lectures on Psycho-Analysis', in *The Standard Edition of the Complete Psychological Works of Sigmund Freud* (London: Hogarth Press, 1933), XXII, 29–30.

[51] Sigmund Freud, 'Moses and Monotheism', in *The Standard Edition of the Complete Psychological Works of Sigmund Freud* (London: Hogarth Press, 1939), XXIII, 68.

a bit of time discussing a particular manifestation of the traumatic neuroses which illustrates how, at least for a brief moment in psychoanalytic history, the relationship between 'external' events and 'internal' psychical processes was taken very seriously. This is the example of the war neuroses.

The Example of the War Neuroses

In September 1918 a Symposium was held at the Fifth International Psycho-Analytical Congress in Budapest on the subject of the war neuroses. Sándor Ferenczi, Karl Abraham and Ernst Simmel all presented papers on this topic, and Freud himself wrote the introduction to the proceedings of the Symposium which were published in *Psycho-Analysis and the War Neuroses* in 1921.[52]

As Pedro Muñoz and Sílvia Correia note in their discussion of the Congress and its significance in the wider context of psychoanalysis in the second decade of the twentieth century, these lectures attracted a great deal of interest from the military and medical authorities representing the Central Powers.[53] And at the time it appeared that a bright future lay ahead for a psychoanalytic understanding of, and a clinical engagement with, the psychical traumas of war. However, it was not to be. Instead, the next sixty years or so saw a progressive disengagement of psychoanalysis from the theory and treatment of the war neuroses, culminating in the disappearance of the term completely from the psychiatric literature and the emergence of a completely new paradigm of trauma in the aftermath of the Vietnam War: post-traumatic stress disorder.

As I note earlier, the term 'war neurosis' (or, more precisely, 'the war neuroses') were regarded by Freud and his colleagues as a form of traumatic neurosis. This is made clear by Freud in his Introduction to the proceedings of the Symposium, and the term 'traumatic neuroses' is used a number of times by both Ferenczi and Abraham in their presentations.

[52] Sándor Ferenczi and others, *Psycho-Analysis and the War Neuroses* (Vienna: The International Psycho-Analytical Press, 1921). The book also included a paper written by Ernest Jones and which was originally read before the Royal Society of Medicine, Section of Psychiatry, in April 1918.

[53] Correia, Sílvia, and Pedro Muñoz, 'The Great War and the Fifth International Psychoanalytic Congress in Budapest: Psychoanalysis in the 1910s', *Historia Crítica*, 84, 2022, 3–27

For example, in his Introduction Freud writes: "The war neuroses, in so far as they differ from the ordinary neuroses of peace time through particular peculiarities, are to be regarded as traumatic neuroses, whose existence has been rendered possible or promoted through an ego-conflict."[54] Somewhat confusingly, perhaps, Freud and Abraham both refer to 'the traumatic neuroses of peace time' but not 'the traumatic neuroses of war (time)', opting instead for the term 'the war neuroses' or simply 'war neurosis'. This might suggest that they are referring to two different phenomena, that is, the traumatic neuroses (of peace) and the war neuroses, but it is clear from their texts that these terms are equivalent. However, this does raise the question as to whether there is something different or extraordinary about the conditions of war as opposed to the conditions of peace which might result in a different form of psychopathology.

One of the dominant themes of the Symposium was to challenge the idea, which was widespread in psychiatric circles, that the war neuroses had 'disproved' Freud's theories, and especially those related to infantile sexuality. To quote Freud again: "…the opponents of psycho-analysis, whose repugnance to sexuality has shown itself to be stronger than their logic, have hastened to proclaim that investigation of the war neuroses has finally disproved this part of the psycho-analytical theory."[55] According to these critics, the psychopathologies that emerged as a result of being shelled, machined gunned, trapped for days or weeks at a time in a trench or dug-out, clearly had nothing to do with childhood Oedipal experiences.

The basic thrust of the argument of all the Symposium's participants, on the other hand, was that the war neuroses were the product of an underlying psychopathology that was rooted in unresolved, childhood sexual conflicts. In other words, those who were suffering from war neurosis were already neurotic.[56] For example, Simmel argued that:

> The psycho-analytical explanation of the war neuroses has proved with wonderful clearness the correctness of the Freudian views on hysteria, according to which all physical symptoms represent conversions of

[54] Ferenczi et al., *Psycho-Analysis and the War Neuroses*, 2.

[55] *Ibid.*, 2.

[56] Or in some cases, psychotic or narcissistic.

> something psychical. The body is the instrument of the mind upon which it (the mind) allows its unconscious to manifest itself in plastic and mimic expression. The functions of the unconscious are the deciding factor in the formation and building up of the war neuroses, also the frequently observed instances of the forgetting of events accompanied by feelings hostile to the ego, even when these events are very recent, permits us to recognise from the outside alone the submergence and repression of ideas and affects of a painful nature.[57]

Ferenczi, Abraham, Jones (in his separate paper) and Freud (in his Introduction) all follow a similar line: the traumatic experiences of war 'trigger' an underlying psychopathology, often hysterical in nature. Just to give one more example, Abraham in somewhat condescending language, argued that: "It transpires with great regularity that the war neurotics already before the trauma were labile people—to designate it, to begin with, by a general expression—and especially so as regards their sexuality."[58] By 'labile' he appears to mean 'emotionally volatile' and which he seems to view as a weakness (in men at least).

On a more general basis, the Great War provided an opportunity for Freud and his colleagues to study the effects of psychical trauma in a relatively controlled environment and on an industrial scale, and to further develop their theory of the neuroses. It also meant, as is often the case in war time, that the medical and military authorities were more open to new and innovative ideas. Muñoz and Correia's note that both Ferenczi and Abraham had had the opportunity to observe traumatised soldiers at close quarters; Ferenczi became head of the department for neurology at the Mária Valéria Military Hospital where he was able to indulge in his interest in the traumatic neuroses, and Abraham became director at the Allenstein Hospital where he was able to observe many cases of war neurosis. Ernst Simmel, the other key contributor at the Budapest Symposium, had been physician in charge at the Military Hospital of Posen where he had gained experience of the war neuroses. So clearly there was already a great deal of interest in the topic within analytic circles.

---

[57] *Ibid.*, 31.

[58] *Ibid.*, 23.

However, and somewhat ironically (as Freud notes in his Introduction), the cessation of hostilities two months after the Congress also put an end to the opportunity to study the war neuroses. What Freud seems to be suggesting here, although he does not elaborate, is that the War was providing an ample supply of 'case material', in hospitals and other health facilities, which could be examined in some detail. Once the War had ended, this 'material' rapidly dissipated, and would probably only to reappear, if at all, many years later in (mainly private) psychoanalytic clinics.

Furthermore, as Muñoz and Correia point out, although the Congress came up with a number of concrete proposals to increase access to psychoanalysis, both for the military and the wider public, as well as appointing Ferenczi as president of the International Psychoanalytic Association (IPA), politics soon intervened in the form of the 'white terror'. This was the overthrow of the communist government of Béla Kun in Hungary by Admiral Miklós Horthy in 1919 who imposed strict antisemitic laws regarding the number of Jewish students and professors at universities. This resulted in Ferenczi, who was himself Jewish, having to relinquish his position to Jones and, perhaps more damaging for psychoanalysis as a whole, meant that many psychoanalysts had to retreat from public life and practice, which was accompanied by the dismantling of the Hungarian Psychoanalytic Association. Clearly, such setbacks did not mean that psychoanalysis as a whole was a doomed enterprise, but they do illustrate how the vagaries of war and politics can have both a positive and negative influence on clinical practice and innovation.[59]

It is also important to note that although psychoanalysis was an important influence in developing the theoretical and clinical understanding of the war neuroses (or 'shell-shock' as it was more popularly known), much of this understanding was decidedly 'un-Freudian', or, if you like,

[59] Although Muñoz and Correia acknowledge that the 'white terror' resulted in the emigration of many analysts (one of the principle reasons for the dismantling of the HPA) they still argue that the Congress had a more lasting legacy; for example in the establishment of free analysis clinics in Berlin, Vienna, London and Tegel. They also highlight the fact that representatives of the military authorities attended the Congress and agreed to open up psychoanalytic treatment stations for soldiers. However, it's important to note that with regards to the latter, this idea never had any real lasting traction.

'Freud-lite'. In other words, although such approaches utilised a number of Freud's concepts, for example that of repression, the unconscious and so on, they also left out or rejected some of the critical aspects of Freud's theory and particularly those relating to the sexual aetiology of the neuroses. For example, one of the most well-known British war psychiatrists, William Halse Rivers Rivers (more commonly known as W H R Rivers) whose most famous patient was probably the war poet Siegfried Sassoon, was a great admirer of Freud's work—but only up to a certain point. This is highlighted in Allan Young's study of Rivers' work where he writes:

> Rivers rejected the theory of infantile sexuality. Where Freud believed that libido and aggression are the primary psychic drives, Rivers emphasized fear and gregariousness. Freud's theory of psychoneurosis was based on a concept of forgetting (repression) that was premised on a dynamic unconscious; Rivers' theory of the unconscious was built on nineteenth-century ideas about dissociation. Stripped of its Jacksonian assumptions, Rivers' theory of forgetting and healing was closer to Pierre Janet's than to Freud's.[60]

It is also interesting to note, as does Ben Shephard, in his study of the war neuroses, that Rivers' relationship with Sassoon, who he treated at the Craiglockhart Hospital in 1917, was problematic in itself.[61] Shephard points out that Sassoon was hardly a typical shell shock patient. In fact, he had been sent to Craiglockhart in order to prevent him from publicising any more of his anti-war views, following his letter in *The Times* questioning the aims of the war. There were added complications, including Rivers' repressed homosexual feelings towards Sassoon, and the fact that Rivers was struggling with his own pacifist views whilst trying to persuade his patients to return to the front. This might raise questions regarding Rivers' real motives for rejecting Freud's ideas about sexuality.

Another example is that of Abram Kardiner, an American doctor who in 1922 began treating ex-soldiers at the No. 81 Veterans' Bureau Hospital in New York City. What was especially interesting about this work is that it was begun four years after the war had ended so even at that time,

60 Allan Young, 'W. H. R. Rivers and the War Neuroses', *Journal of the History of the Behavioral Sciences*, 35.4 (1999), 359–78, 372.

61 Shephard, *A War of Nerves*.

many decades before the advent of PTSD, it was clear that the psychological effects of war were enduring. Kardiner spent four years at the Hospital and out of the 700 he had diagnosed as having traumatic neuroses he treated around 150 and eventually published 24 case studies. It is also important to note that Kardiner had been in analysis with Freud himself immediately after the war—and yet as Shephard points out, the more he tried to apply the key Freudian concepts to his patients, especially relating to libido theory, the less relevant they seemed:

> If anything, his material—with its recurrent motif of the man paralysed or rendered unconscious by a sensory stimulus—pointed in a different direction altogether, towards the work of the Russian psychologist Pavlov and of Pavlov's American affiliates, the behavioural psychiatrists.[62]

Ironically, perhaps, Kardiner's ideas were finally published in book form in 1941, just as the United States was about to enter another world war.[63] By this point Kardiner's view of the war neuroses were very far removed from Freud's. Rather than events 'triggering' an underlying psychopathology, which had its roots in infantile sexual conflicts, Kardiner was arguing a neurosis was rooted in an inability of the subject to adapt to a new environment, which is caused by the 'trauma' of the event. As Shephard comments, there was something of a paradox when it came to the publication of Kardiner's book: by that time very few in the psychiatric profession in the United States and in Britain were interested in his ideas:

> And yet, ultimately Kardiner would prove the most influential writer on the war neuroses. In the 1970s, when American medicine was confronted by an epidemic of mental disorders in Vietnam veterans, his book was a bible, almost the only thing the psychiatrist could turn to.[64]

But this would be a 'bible' devoid of the key scripture of its (and Kardiner's) master, Freud.

---

[62] *Ibid.*, 155.

[63] Abram Kardiner, *The Traumatic Neuroses of War* (Eastford, Connecticut: Martino Fine Books, 2012).

[64] Shephard, *A War of Nerves*, 157.

'Traumatic' or 'Actual' Neuroses?

As I indicated earlier, there is some debate as to whether the traumatic neuroses might belong to a completely different 'category' of psychopathology than that of the psychoneuroses, namely the *actual neuroses*. The fact that the traumatic neuroses appear to be caused by events in the present or near present seems to undermine the idea that these might be linked to childhood sexual conflicts that have been subjected to repression and other psychical operations. It then appears to be a short step to arguing that this means that a traumatic neurosis is, in fact, an actual neurosis. My contention, however, is that, in fact, the reverse is the case, that is, an actual neurosis is another term for a traumatic one. But before making this case it is necessary to gain a better understanding of what Freud meant by the term 'actual neurosis'.

In the Drafts B and E of the *Fliess papers*, Freud raises the question of the actual neuroses for the first time, although he does not use the term explicitly. In Draft B he discusses in some detail the sexual aetiology of neurasthenia and anxiety neurosis, with a specific focus on how neurasthenia varies between males and females. In males Freud argues that this is often acquired at puberty, appears in the subject's twenties, and its source is masturbation. In older males it can be caused by attempts by the male subject to avoid conception. Young females, according to Freud, tend not to suffer from neurasthenia. In the rare cases where neurasthenia arises in married women and older unmarried ones, Freud argues that this arises in the same manner as it does in men (though he does not explicitly state what he means by this). More often, he argues: "…neurasthenia in a married woman is derived from neurasthenia in a man or is produced simultaneously. In that case there is almost always an admixture of hysteria and we have the common mixed neurosis of women."[65] He ends his text by stating that such neuroses are both "entirely preventable as well as entirely incurable."[66]

[65] Freud, *The Complete Letters*, 42.

[66] *Ibid.*, 43.

In Draft E Freud focuses on anxiety neurosis and concludes that this is the result of a physical sexual tension (excitation) arising internally which is not able to be transformed into a psychical tension:

> The physical tension increases, reaches the threshold value at which it can arouse psychical affect; but for some reasons the psychical linkage offered to it remains insufficient: a *sexual affect* cannot be formed, because there is something lacking in the psychical determinants. Accordingly, the physical tension, not being psychically bound, is transformed into—anxiety.[67]

It is worth noting here that what Freud appears to be suggesting is that the actual neuroses are rooted in libidinal excitation, which Lacan will come to define as jouissance.

In his paper *Sexuality in the Aetiology of the Neuroses* Freud discusses the difference between neurasthenia and the psychoneuroses with regards to the sexual aetiology of the neuroses: "Thus, in every case of neurosis there is a sexual aetiology; but in neurasthenia it is an aetiology of a present-day kind, whereas in the psychoneuroses the factors are of an infantile nature."[68] He further 'breaks down' neurasthenia into 'neurasthenia proper' and anxiety neurosis and argues that the former is where symptoms such as intracranial pressure, fatigue, constipation, etc. are prominent, and with the latter such symptoms only play a minor part and "…the clinical picture is composed of other symptoms, all of which exhibit a relation to the nuclear symptom, that of anxiety…"[69] Later on in the paper Freud uses the term 'actual neuroses' explicitly for the first time:

> The value of making a correct diagnostic separation of the psychoneuroses from neurasthenia is also shown by the fact that the psychoneuroses call for a different practical assessment and for special therapeutic measures. They make their appearance as a result of two kinds of determinants, either independently or in the train of the 'actual neuroses' (neurasthenia and anxiety neurosis).[70]

[67] *Ibid.*, 80–81, italics in original.

[68] Sigmund Freud, 'Sexuality in the Aetiology of the Neuroses', in *The Standard Edition of the Complete Psychological Works of Sigmund Freud* (London: Hogarth Press, 1898), III, 268.

[69] *Ibid.*, 268.

[70] *Ibid.*, 278–279. However, Strachey points out that the concept is implied in Freud's earlier works, for example in *Studies on Hysteria*.

The last sentence is particularly interesting because this is something Freud will return to some eighteen years later (see below) and is the idea that an actual neurosis can form the basis of a psychoneurosis.

In lecture 24 of his *Introductory Lectures* Freud gives quite a comprehensive summary of his theory of the actual neuroses, some twenty years after he originally formulated the idea. However, he also goes further and argues that the actual neuroses are a consequence of the *somatic* dimension of sexual disturbances. In fact, he even goes so far as to argue that such neuroses are the result of some form of 'sexual toxicity' in the body:

> The 'actual' neuroses, in the details of their symptoms and also their characteristic of influencing every organic system and every function, exhibit an unmistakable resemblance to the pathological states which arise from the chronic influence of external toxic substances and from a sudden withdrawal of them—to intoxications and conditions of abstinence … In view of these analogies, we cannot, I think, avoid regarding the neuroses as results of disturbances in the sexual metabolism, whether because more of these sexual toxins is produced than the subject can deal with, or whether because internal and even psychical conditions restrict the proper employment of these substances.[71]

What Freud seems to be hinting at here, although using different terminology, is the idea that the actual neuroses (neurasthenia and anxiety neurosis[72]) are linked to what later on in this work I describe as the *jouissance of the drive.* If by 'sexual toxins', which Freud admits is an analogy, he really means libidinal excitation, then it seems reasonable to argue that what Freud describes as "disturbances in the sexual metabolism" is actually the trauma of the drive, that is, the excess excitation of the drive, which I have defined as drive-jouissance. If this is the case then it sheds a different light on Freud's argument later on in the same lecture, and which I touched on earlier, that symptoms of an actual neurosis can provide the nucleus for a psychoneurosis:

---

[71] Freud, 'Introductory Lectures', 338.

[72] Laplanche and Pontalis note that later on Freud also proposed that hypochondria should be included amongst the actual neuroses.

> Let us take as an example a case of hysterical headache or lumbar pain. Analysis shows us that, by condensation and displacement, it has become a substitutive satisfaction for a whole number of libidinal phantasies or memories. But this pain was also at one time a real one and it was then a direct sexual-toxic symptom, the somatic expression of a libidinal excitation.[73]

Regarding the 'actuality' in the actual neuroses, Laplanche and Pontalis point out that:

> The opposition between the actual neuroses and the psychoneuroses is essentially aetiological and pathogenic: the cause is definitely sexual in both these types of neurosis, but in the former case it must be sought in a disorder of [the subject's] contemporary sexual life' and not in 'important events in his past life'. The adjective 'actual' is therefore to be understood first and foremost in the sense of *temporal* 'actuality'.[74]

The key point here is that in the actual neuroses the memory of the 'traumatic' event has not undergone repression or any form of psychical working over. This is why Freud argued that such neuroses were incurable, that is, not amenable to psychoanalysis. But in my view there is also a tendency to conflate or confuse *temporality* with *externality*. Freud is *not* arguing that the causes of the actual neuroses lie in the 'external' world; on the contrary he is clear they relate to 'internal', biological processes which, for reasons that Freud is still not very clear about, have 'bypassed' psychical mediation.

It is important to note that there is nothing in Freud's theory of the actual neuroses that *precludes* the existence of a psychoneurosis as well. In the *Introductory Lecture* I cited earlier Freud argues that an actual neurosis can provide the nucleus for a psychoneurosis. But couldn't it equally be argued that a psychoneuroses provides the nucleus for an actual neurosis? The example that Freud uses, the hysterical headache, could well be a "substitutive satisfaction for a whole number of libidinal phantasies or memories". At the same time, though, Freud is arguing that at some

[73] *Ibid.*, 390–391.

[74] Laplanche and Pontalis, *The Language of Psychoanalysis*, 10.

point in the subject's history this pain was "the somatic expression of a libidinal excitation". But such an expression of a libidinal excitation sounds suspiciously like the excitation produced by the drive, which later on in this work I will define as drive-jouissance. So, is it possible that what Freud describes as the 'actual neuroses' are the *effect* of drive-jouissance, not the *cause*?

But to what extent do the *actual* neuroses differ from the *traumatic* ones? In their 2007 paper on actual neurosis Paul Verhaeghe, Stijn Vanheule and Ann De Rick argue that a range of pathologies, including panic, somatic and undifferentiated disorders can all be reclassified as forms of actual neurosis.[75] These ideas are summarised in a lecture that Verhaeghe gave in Dublin in 2008 where he proposes the term 'actual pathology' to encompass a range of pathologies that do not fit into the 'classical' Freudian category of the psychoneuroses.[76] Such pathologies have symptomatologies that bring the somatic dimension of the subject's experience to the fore, for example through self-mutilation and eating disorders and a range of psychosomatic conditions.[77] Furthermore, such symptomatologies lack meaning and cannot (apparently) be situated within the subject's history. Crucially, in the same lecture Verhaeghe argues that the traumatic neuroses should also be included within the category of actual pathologies. In a previous 2005 paper, Verhaeghe and Vanheule had argued that PTSD could also be seen as an example of an actual neurosis because of the centrality of anxiety and somatisation in the symptomatology of PTSD.[78] And in that paper the authors also emphasised the importan of the Other (or rather its *absence* in the case of actual pathologies) in laying down the foundations for psychical mediation for the infant subject and particularly in relation to the regulation of the drive:

---

[75] Paul Verhaeghe, Stijn Vanheule, and Ann De Rick, "Actual Neurosis as the Underlying Psychic Structure of Panic Disorder, Somatization, and Somatoform Disorder: An Integration of Freudian and Attachment Perspectives," *The Psychoanalytic Quarterly* 76, no. 4 (October 1, 2007): 1317–50.

[76] Paul Verhaeghe, "A Combination That Has to Fail: New Patients, Old Therapists.," *Eisteach (Dun Laoghaire)* 8, no. 4 (2008): 4–8.

[77] The latter should not be confused with the 'classic' conversion symptoms, for example in cases of hysteria.

[78] Paul Verhaeghe and Stijn Vanheule, "Actual Neurosis and PTSD: The Impact of the Other," *Psychoanalytic Psychology* 22, no. 4 (2005): 493–507.

> Joining Freud's theory of the development of the ego to his distinction between actual neurosis and psychoneurosis, we can outline the impact of the Other in this distinction much more clearly. In the case of a psychoneurotic development, the pressure resulting from the drive is processed via the mirroring reaction of the Other. On these grounds, the subject acquires a representational identity, a "theory of the mind," whose further oedipal elaboration may lead to the construction of meaningful symptoms based on unconscious fantasies. This transforms the original automatic anxiety into a defensive signal anxiety. The nature of the symptoms will be determined by the specific mechanisms of defense. In case of an actual neurosis, however, the elaboration does not occur; the subject remains stuck in this transition. The effect with regard to the clinical picture of actual neurosis is an absence of "meaningful" symptoms and the preponderance of anxiety-related somatic phenomena, these being expressions of the automatic anxiety.[79]

Whilst in this paper Verhaeghe and Vanheule are using the Lacanian concept of the Other, particular in its role in the mirror stage, to explain the concept of psychical mediation, in the subsequent 2007 paper all references to Lacan mysteriously disappear and are replaced by references to attachment theory and the importance of the primary caregiver in alleviating the primordial anxiety that the infant experiences.[80] Be that as it may, what is really at stake here is the authors' argument for a separate category of 'actual pathology'. Although I believe they are correct, along with many other psychoanalytic theorists and practitioners, to highlight the emergence over the last few decades of a range of pathologies that cannot readily be classified as (psycho) neurosis, psychosis or perversion (the three 'classical' clinical structures), my contention is that subsuming these all under the heading of 'actual pathology' or 'actual neurosis' is

---

[79] *Ibid.*, 501.

[80] Although even in the 2005 paper the concept of the 'Other' is being used somewhat ambiguously by the authors. Strictly speaking, if they are referring to the role of the mother or other primary caregiver in 'mediating' the effect of the drive and the resulting anxiety in the infant, then the term 'other' (with a small o) should be used, because the 'Other' refers to the Symbolic order and the unconscious—although it should be noted that this 'big Other' plays a key role in the mirror stage as formulated by Lacan.

unhelpful.[81] Indeed, I think there is strong case for such pathologies to be incorporated within the category of traumatic neurosis instead.

The primary reason I argue this is that it follows Freud's own trajectory of thought. In his 1925 autobiographical paper Freud makes reference to his theory of the actual neuroses and that he regarded them as "…the direct toxic expression of such disturbances [of the sexual function]…"[82] This is clearly in line with his discussions of the actual neuroses that I highlighted earlier in this chapter. However, he then goes on to state:

> Since that time I have had no opportunity of returning to the investigation of the 'actual neuroses', nor has this part of my work been continued by anyone else. If I look back to-day at my early findings, they strike me as being the first rough outlines of what is probably a far more complicated subject.[83]

Although, just to complicate things even more, Freud then goes on to state that:

> But on the whole they seem to me still to hold good … I should like to make it clear that I am far from denying the existence of mental conflicts and of neurotic complexes in neurasthenia. All that I am asserting is that the symptoms of these patients are not mentally determined or removed by analysis, but they must be regarded as direct toxic consequences of disturbed sexual chemical processes.[84]

It's hard to see how Freud can argue on the one hand that his arguments regarding the actual neuroses still 'hold good' and yet on the other hand he acknowledges that neither he nor anyone else had had the opportunity to explore this topic further in recent years! What *is* clear, however, in a key text that Freud published a year later, namely *Inhibitions, Symptoms and Anxiety* and which I referred to earlier in this chapter, is that he

[81] Although in his Dublin lecture Verhaeghe uses the term 'actual pathology, in both his 2005 and 2007 papers he refers to 'actual neurosis' and these appear to be referring to the same thing.

[82] Sigmund Freud, "An Autobiographical Study," in *The Standard Edition of the Complete Psychological Works of Sigmund Freud*, vol. XX (London: Hogarth Press, 1925), 25.

[83] *Ibid.*, 26.

[84] *Ibid.*, 26.

significantly changed his view on the nature of one of the key aspects of the actual neuroses: anxiety. Whereas in previous writings Freud had argued that anxiety is rooted in the libido he now argued that it is rooted in the ego and is a response to a perceived danger, for example, castration. As I noted earlier, it is also in this paper that Freud argues that trauma is the source of anxiety for the subject, which may be 'external' or 'internal'—in the latter case this trauma is emanating from the drive. In fact, strictly speaking by this point in Freud's work on trauma, it is only the 'internal' danger that is truly 'traumatic':

> So far we have had no occasion to regard realistic anxiety in any different light from neurotic anxiety. We [now?] know what the distinction is. A real danger is a danger which threatens a person from an external object, and a neurotic danger is one which threatens him from an instinctual [drive] demand. In so far as the instinctual demand is something real, his neurotic anxiety, too, can be admitted to have a realistic basis.[85]

In my view Freud's arguments regarding anxiety in this paper represent a subtle and yet significant shift in his thinking. On the one hand he is still arguing that the drive is a source of anxiety for the subject; and yet on the other hand he is arguing that this is a response from the *ego*. As I understand it, in his previous writings Freud was essentially arguing that anxiety resided in the excitation of the drive itself; in other words, it was a *somatic* effect. Now he is arguing that anxiety is the ego's *response* to the excitation of the drive. This shift in Freud's thinking matters because it is the *subject* that is traumatised not the *drive*. If the anxiety is in the drive itself then it makes no sense to speak of the drive as 'traumatising' or 'wounding'. Furthermore, the concept of *trauma* now takes centre stage and the 'actuality' of the libidinal excitation is, in many ways, inconsequential. What I mean by this is that it is not the temporality of the trauma that matters to the subject but its 'wounding' nature. In fact, and as I discuss in some length in Chap. 6, the whole concept of 'actuality', that is, occurring in the here-and-now, is itself deeply problematic because of Freud's idea of *Nachträglichkeit*.

[85] Freud, *Inhibitions, Symptoms and Anxiety*, 167.

At the same time I think it is important to remember that Freud retained the idea of the traumatic neuroses right until the end, whereas he seems to have, to all intents and purposes, abandoned the idea of the actual neuroses pretty much mid-way through his analytic career (the time of the *Introductory Lectures).* And this leads me back to my central assertion regarding the actual neuroses: the idea essentially becomes redundant in Freud's work because his concept of the traumatic neuroses supersedes it, particularly by the time of *Inhibitions, Symptoms and Anxiety*. The reason Freud needed the concept of the actual neuroses in his earlier work, I would argue, is because at that time he still hadn't properly differentiated the traumatic neuroses from the psychoneuroses. By the time of *Beyond the Pleasure Principle*, however, this differentiation becomes much clearer. If the trauma in question is the excitation of the drive (which in this book I refer to as drive-jouissance) then this accounts for the somatic nature of the so-called actual neuroses and is equally applicable to the traumatic neuroses.

Although in some ways it might seem a matter of semantics whether the term 'actual' or 'traumatic' is used, in this case, I would argue, semantics matter a great deal. The 'traumatic' in traumatic neurosis shifts the emphasis to the wounding effect of the drive on the subject; the 'actual' in actual neurosis shifts the emphasis to the 'here-and-now' of the subject's experience of … the trauma of the drive, whilst essentially circumventing the problematic questions of the temporality and historisation of such trauma, and the role that psychoanalysis might have in confronting such questions.

However, before pursuing such questions in this work, I now want to turn to another question. As I briefly discussed earlier, one of Freud's arguments in *Beyond the Pleasure Principle* was that the traumatic excitations that breached the subject's psychical defences put the pleasure principle out of action. In terms of how my arguments regarding trauma and the traumatic neuroses unfold in this book, the concept of the pleasure principle and its vicissitudes is absolutely fundamental, so it is to this topic that we must now turn.

3

The Pleasure Principle and Its Vicissitudes: From Psychophysics to Cybernetics

Introduction

As I pointed out in the previous chapter, one of Freud's arguments in *Beyond the Pleasure Principle* regarding trauma was that it disabled the pleasure principle. But what exactly does Freud mean by the pleasure principle and what role does it have in regulating excitation, which he links to trauma? Furthermore, how does Lacan approach this concept within the framework of language? In this chapter I will explore in some depth the concept of the pleasure principle and its close relation to the principle of constancy. I will begin by discussing Freud's formulation of these two concepts and then outline Laplanche's attempt to address some of the contradictions that arise in Freud's approach to these ideas and particularly what often appears to be a conflation of the pleasure principle and the principle of constancy. I will then discuss Lacan's approach to the pleasure principle with a particular focus on his arguments in *Seminar II* regarding the relationship of the pleasure principle to language, cybernetics and the death drive. I conclude the chapter with a brief discussion of the impact of 'French Theory' on subsequent readings of Lacan's work.

© The Author(s), under exclusive license to Springer Nature Switzerland AG 2025

L. Chapman, *Traumatic Neurosis Revisited*, The Palgrave Lacan Series,
https://doi.org/10.1007/978-3-031-89158-8_3

Freud's Theory of the Pleasure Principle

In their discussion of the pleasure principle in *The Language of Psychoanalysis,* Laplanche and Pontalis note that it is an idea that remains broadly unchanged throughout Freud's work.[1] However, it is the relationship to other key concepts, and especially the reality principle and principle of constancy, that remains problematic. One of the key issues is whether the pleasure principle aims to maintain a constant level of energy in the psychical apparatus or to reduce it to a minimum level.

In chapter VII, section D, of *The Interpretation of Dreams* Freud discusses arousal by dreams, the function of dreams and anxiety-dreams. In the first part he explores the path of unconscious wishes as they attempt to reach consciousness, in a distorted form, but are blocked by the sleeping state of the preconscious. Such wishes evade this barrier by becoming visual representations:

> The dream-process consequently enters on a regressive path, which lies open to it precisely owing to the peculiar nature of the state of sleep, and it is led along that path by the attraction exercised on it by groups of memories; some of these memories themselves exist only in the form of visual cathexes and not as translations into the terminology of the later systems. In the course of its regressive path the dream-process acquires the attribute of representability.[2]

Freud then makes reference to consciousness, as a sense organ, receiving (in waking life) excitations from two directions: the perceptual system and pleasure/unpleasure. The latter Freud identifies as emanating from within the psyche and states: "We are thus driven to conclude that *these releases of pleasure and unpleasure automatically regulate the course of the cathectic processes*."[3] Freud goes onto to argue that every dream has an arousing effect "…that it sets a part of the quiescent force of the Pcs. in action. The dream is then submitted by this force to the influence which

[1] Laplanche and Pontalis, *The Language of Psychoanalysis*, 322–325.

[2] Sigmund Freud, 'The Interpretation of Dreams (Second Part)', in *The Standard Edition of the Complete Psychological Works of Sigmund Freud* (London: Hogarth Press, 1900), V, 573–574.

[3] *Ibid.*, 574, italics in original.

we have described as secondary revision with an eye to consecutiveness and intelligibility."[4]

With regards to the pleasure principle, which in this text Freud refers to as the *unpleasure* principle, he discusses this in the context of the flow of excitatory material into consciousness (*Cs.*). Freud argues that this can originate from the *Pcpt.* system and from the interior of the psychical apparatus itself "...whose quantitative processes are felt qualitatively in the pleasure-unpleasure series when, subject to certain modifications, they make their way to consciousness."[5] Consciousness, according to Freud, functions to regulate the flow of excitatory material:

> By perceiving new qualities, it (Cs.) makes a new contribution to directing the mobile quantities of cathexis and distributing them in an expedient fashion. By the help of its perception of pleasure and unpleasure it influences the discharge of cathexes within what is otherwise an unconscious apparatus operating by means of the displacement of quantities.[6]

Freud suggests that whilst in the first instance the (un)pleasure principle regulates the discharge of the cathexes automatically, consciousness 'perfects' this process. These remarks indicate that even in his earlier writings Freud was recognising that some excitations originated from 'within' the psyche, although he does not specifically mention the drives. Whereas in *Beyond the Pleasure Principle* he emphasises the 'external' nature of such excitations, in *The Interpretation of Dreams* Freud also emphasises that dreams can be seen as a form of expression of underlying 'impulses' "...which are under the pressure of resistance during the day but which have been able to find reinforcement during the night from deep-lying sources of excitation."[7]

In *Instincts and their Vicissitudes* Freud references the pleasure principle in the context of his discussion of the operation of the drives ('instincts' in the Standard Edition) and how they make greater demands on the psychical apparatus than external stimuli:

---

[4] *Ibid.*, 575.

[5] *Ibid.*, 616

[6] *Ibid.*, 616.

[7] *Ibid.*, 614.

> External stimuli impose only the single task of withdrawing from them; this is accomplished by muscular movements, one of which eventually achieves that aim and thereafter, being the expedient movement, becomes a hereditary disposition. Instinctual stimuli, which originate from within the organism, cannot be dealt with by this mechanism. Thus they make far higher demands on the nervous system and cause it to undertake involved and interconnected activities by which the external world is so changed as to afford satisfaction to the internal source of stimulation.[8]

Freud goes onto to suggest that the drives are the "true motive force" that have led to the development of the nervous system (psychical apparatus). He then refers to the pleasure principle as regulating the activity of the psychical apparatus "…i.e. is automatically regulated by feelings belonging to the pleasure-unpleasure series…" and therefore:

> …we can hardly reject the further hypothesis that these feelings reflect the manner in which the process of mastering stimuli takes place—certainly in the sense that unpleasurable feelings are connected with an increase and pleasurable feelings with a decrease of stimulus."[9]

What's particularly interesting here, in my view, is that Freud is already emphasising, five years before *Beyond the Pleasure Principle*, that the drives are an important source of 'stimulation' (excitation). Furthermore, the drives are a *constant force*, unlike external stimuli, which is what makes the role of the pleasure principle so crucial. In other words, the drives are producing a constant jouissance in the subject, which needs to be regulated.

In *The Economic Problem of Masochism* Freud gives a useful summary and clarification of his idea of the pleasure principle in relation to the principle of constancy and the idea of the 'Nirvana principle', which he takes from Barbara Low. In fact, as Strachey points out in a footnote on page 159, in his text Freud is using the term 'Nirvana principle' in place of the principle of constancy, which he used in *Beyond the Pleasure Principle*. Freud argues that the pleasure principle is a 'special case' of the principle of constancy. He then states that:

---

[8] Sigmund Freud, 'Instincts and Their Vicissitudes', in *The Standard Edition of the Complete Psychological Works of Sigmund Freud* (London: Hogarth Press, 1915), XIV, 120.

[9] *Ibid.*, 120–121.

> ...we have unhesitatingly identified the pleasure-unpleasure principle with the Nirvana principle. Every unpleasure ought thus to coincide with a heightening, and every pleasure with a lowering, of mental tension due to stimulus; the Nirvana principle (and the pleasure principle which is supposedly identical with it) would be entirely in the service of the death instincts, whose aim is to conduct the restlessness of life into the stability of the inorganic state...[10]

However, at this point Freud argues that such a view is wrong. He notes that not all pleasurable experiences are experienced as a *reduction* in tension, and not all unpleasurable ones are experienced as an *increase* in tension. He cites sexual pleasure as an example of the former, although he does not give an example of the latter. This leads Freud to conclude that pleasure and unpleasure cannot be viewed in *quantitative* terms (as an increase or decrease in tension). Rather, they depend on some (unidentified) *qualitative* factor. Freud then goes onto argue that:

> ...we must perceive that the Nirvana principle, belonging as it does to the death instinct, has undergone a modification in living organisms through which it has become the pleasure principle; and we shall henceforward avoid regarding the two principles as one ... The *Nirvana* principle expresses the trend of the death instinct; the *pleasure* principle represents the demands of the libido; and the modification of the latter principle, the *reality* principle, represents the influence of the external world.[11]

Perhaps another way to express this is to argue that the pleasure principle is the *regulation* of libido (which Lacan will later redefine as jouissance). This would mean that the pleasure principle is essentially the same as the principle of constancy—something I will be exploring shortly. Freud concludes that the pleasure principle, the Nirvana principle and the reality principle are able to 'tolerate' one another 'as a rule'. He then states:

---

[10] Sigmund Freud, 'The Economic Problem of Masochism', in *The Standard Edition of the Complete Psychological Works of Sigmund Freud* (London: Hogarth Press, 1924), XIX, 159–160.

[11] *Ibid.*, 160, italics in original.

"The conclusion to be drawn from these considerations is that the descriptions of the pleasure principle as the watchman over our life cannot be rejected."[12]

The Principle of Constancy

The metaphor of the watchman seems to reinforce the idea that Freud saw the pleasure principle, at least in some of his writings, as a *regulatory* principle. However, the concept of regulation, which in this case refers to the regulation of psychical energy, immediately brings up the question of *constancy*, which is the idea that the 'regulation' of the psychical apparatus refers to the level of energy (excitation) being kept at a constant level. And one of the difficulties with Freud's concept of the pleasure principle, which I have already alluded to, is that there appears to be a great deal of ambiguity as to whether he regards it as a principle of constancy or, more radically, a 'principle of zero', whereby the psychical apparatus aims to reduce excitation to a 'zero' or 'null' state. In this case, as I noted in the previous section, the pleasure principle becomes equated with the Nirvana principle and the death drive.

The first recorded mention of the concept of the principle of constancy in Freud's work (although not referred to as such) is in Sketch A of his *Sketches for the 'Preliminary Communication' of 1893.*[13] It appears as a brief note in his letter to Breuer on 29 June 1892 (Sketch A) and is stated fully in 'On the Theory of Hysterical Attacks' (Sketch C) where Freud writes:

> *The nervous system endeavours to keep constant something in its functional relational relations that we may describe as the 'sum of excitation'. It puts this precondition of health into effect by disposing associatively of every sensible accretion of excitation or by discharging it by an appropriate motor reaction.*[14]

[12] *Ibid.*, 161.

[13] Sigmund Freud, "Sketches for the 'Preliminary Communication' of 1893," in *The Standard Edition of the Complete Psychological Works of Sigmund Freud*, vol. I (London: Hogarth Press, 1940–1941), 147–54.

[14] Sigmund Freud, 'Sketches for the "Preliminary Communication" of 1893', in *The Standard Edition of the Complete Psychological Works of Sigmund Freud* (London: Hogarth Press, 1940–1941), I, 153–154, italics in original.

Freud goes onto argue that hysterical attacks occur when the psychical impressions that accompany such excitations fail to find adequate discharge, either because the subject refuses to deal with them "...for fear of distressing mental conflicts..." or because they are "...forbidden to do so by modesty or social conditions..." (especially if such impressions are of a sexual nature), or because the subject has received such impressions "...in a state in which his nervous system was incapable of fulfilling the task of disposing of them."[15] And perhaps most importantly of all this leads Freud to define psychical trauma as "*...any impression which the nervous system has difficulty in disposing of by means of associative thinking or of motor reaction...*"[16] What is particularly striking here is the fact that Freud has already sketched out his theory of trauma (and, in effect, traumatic neurosis) nearly thirty years before his discussion of the same topic in *Beyond the Pleasure Principle.*

In his *Project for a Scientific Psychology* Freud discusses the flow of energy in the psychical apparatus (*Q*)[17] and the principle of neuronal inertia, that is, the tendency of neurones to discharge energy (*Q*).[18] As Strachey points out in a footnote, this will later become referred to by Freud as the principle of constancy. Freud argues that such a neuronal discharge is the main function of the nervous system and that "...among the paths of discharge those are preferred and retained which involve a cessation of the stimulus: *flight from the stimulus.*"[19] He then goes onto to note that: "With an [increasing] complexity of the interior [of the organism], the nervous system receives stimuli from the somatic element itself—endogenous stimuli—which have equally to be discharged."[20] This is essentially prefiguring Freud's argument in *Beyond the Pleasure Principle* and *Inhibitions, Symptoms and Anxiety*, that the excitations arising from the drives cannot be dealt with through (physical) flight. However, Freud then proceeds to develop a rather complex argument regarding the relationship between such 'internal' (endogenous) excitations and those

[15] *Ibid.*, 154.
[16] *Ibid.*, 154, italics in original.
[17] Which Freud also refers to as *Qṅ* (for a useful discussion of *Q* see Appendix C of the text).
[18] Freud, 'Project for a Scientific Psychology'. See especially pp. 295–297.
[19] *Ibid.*, 296, italics in original.
[20] *Ibid.*, 297.

emanating from the external world. The crux of his argument is that the 'endogenous' stimuli (those emanating from the drives) are linked to needs of the organism (he cites hunger, respiration and sex as three examples). With regards to how the organism responds to such endogenous stimuli, Freud argues that it can no longer rely on the original principle of inertia, which is to reduce the level of energy to zero. Rather:

> It must put up with [maintaining] a store of *Qὴ* sufficient to meet the demand for a specific action. Nevertheless, the manner in which it does this shows that the same trend persists, modified into an endeavour at least to keep the *Qὴ* as low as possible and to guard against any increase of it—that is, to keep it constant. All functions of the nervous system can be comprised either under the aspect of the primary function or of the secondary one imposed by the exigencies of life.[21]

The primary function that Freud refers to here is that of neuronal discharge in response to external stimuli; the secondary one refers to the response of the organism to excitation of the drives, which in turn are responding to the demands (exigencies) of life. What is important here with regards to the principle of constancy is Freud's idea that although the endogenous excitations cannot be reduced to zero (the death drive not withstanding), they can be maintained at a (relatively) low and constant level. This ensures the survival of the organism without it being overwhelmed by the excitations (trauma) of the drives.

The principle of constancy reappears a number of times in Freud's later works, for example in *Instincts and their Vicissitudes* where he argues that the excitation of drives is the true motivating force that has led to advances in the nervous system in order to prevent the psychical apparatus being overwhelmed. And in *Beyond the Pleasure Principle* he argues that: "The dominating tendency of mental life … is the effort to reduce, to keep constant or to remove internal tension due to stimuli (the 'Nirvana Principle' to borrow a term from Barbara Low)—a tendency which finds expression in the pleasure principle…"[22] At this point, however, it is

[21] *Ibid.*, 297.

[22] *Ibid.*, Freud, 'Beyond the Pleasure Principle', 55–56.

already clear that the ambiguity I referred to earlier in Freud's writing regarding the relationship between the pleasure principle and the principle of constancy is becoming a problem. This is because by the time he gets to write *The Economic Problem of Masochism* he is essentially arguing that the pleasure principle equates with the principle of constancy and functions to regulate libido. By this point, the Nirvana principle has become an operation of the death drive.

At this juncture it is worth noting that much of Freud's thinking around the idea of the principle of constancy (and by extension, the pleasure principle) was heavily influenced by nineteenth century psychophysics and especially the writings of Gustav Fechner, who was also an important influence on the work of William James. Stephanie Hawkins, in her study of James and Fechner, explains that Fechner can be regarded as the founder of psychophysics and used the term to describe the relationship between physiological processes that accompanied psychical events.[23] Hawkins also notes that some of Fechner's and James' ideas have been influential in modern neurobiological thinking. However, it is critical to point out that Fechner was *not* arguing that psychical events could be 'reduced' to physiological processes; rather:

> For Fechner, the psychical (or mental) and the physical (or material) were different modalities of experience. Like the opposing sides of a single coin, the psychical and the physical were functionally parallel; they operated simultaneously, yet maintained an interdependency that was not linked by causality.[24]

Henri Ellenberger argues that Freud acknowledged his debt to Fechner in many instances.[25] This is in spite of the fact that Fechner had a much more spiritual and metaphysical focus than Freud, including a belief in God and life after death. Fechner's concept of the pleasure principle was originally formulated in his book *On the Highest Good*.[26] As Ellenberger

[23] Stephanie Hawkins, "William James, Gustav Fechner, and Early Psychophysics," *Frontiers in Physiology* 2 (2011).

[24] *Ibid.*, 2.

[25] Henri Ellenberger, "Fechner and Freud," *Bulletin of the Menninger Clinic* 20, no. 4 (1956): 201–14.

[26] *Über das höchste Gut*, Leipzig, Breitkopf & Härtel, 1846. I have been unable to identify any English translations of Fechner's texts, so I have relied on Ellenberger's summary of their key points and the original German references.

notes, the Freudian principle of pleasure-unpleasure "...may be considered as a late development of an old concept, which under the name of hedonism, played an important role in the history of philosophy, from Epicurus and Aristippus to Jeremy Bentham and Adam Smith."[27] However, with Fechner this idea takes a completely new turn because he argues that human beings do not seek as it is in reality but what in the subject's conscious or unconscious experience is associated with the *representation* of pleasure. In other words, for Fechner there is no 'innate' sense of what is pleasurable or unpleasurable.

Fechner also developed his own version of the principle of constancy, which he formulated in terms of a principle of stability.[28] For Fechner this reached far beyond a psychological or psycho-biological process of homeostasis but rather was "...a universal principle with which he could supplement the principle of causality in order to give a satisfactory explanation of the universe."[29] As Ellenberger notes, Freud (in *Beyond the Pleasure Principle*) regarded the principle of constancy as a particular case of Fechner's more general principle of stability. Furthermore, he (Freud) also argued that the pleasure principle followed from the principle of constancy: "...actually the latter principle was inferred from the facts which forced us to adopt the pleasure principle."[30]

Beyond the Pleasure Principle

So far, my focus has been on exploring Freud's theory of the pleasure principle and how it relates to the principle of constancy, and already it can be seen that there are some difficulties with the two concepts, and especially how one relates to the other. However, before discussing such problems in more detail, I need to address another key element of Freud's

---

[27] *Ibid.*, 209.

[28] *Einige Ideen zur Schöpfungs und Entwickelungsechichte der Organismen*, Leipzig, Breitkopf & Härtel, 1873.

[29] Ellenberger, 'Fechner and Freud', 211. Ellenberger points out that, according to Fechner, the 'principle of stability' was first used by Zöllner, the German astronomer, as part of his theory of sunspots and the movement of comets.

[30] Freud, 'Beyond the Pleasure Principle', 9.

theory, which is the question of failure or break down of the pleasure principle. I am referring here to Freud's concept of the death drive, which he introduces in *Beyond the Pleasure Principle*. As a number of commentators have pointed out, Freud's theory of the death drive was at the time, and still remains, highly controversial. For example, Richard Boothby argues that Freud's theory of the death drive "...is arguably the darkest and most stubborn riddle posed by the legacy of psychoanalysis."[31] As Boothby goes onto point out, many psychoanalysts have since dismissed the idea as pseudo-science, although analysts such as Jean Laplanche, Melanie Klein and Lacan himself took it very seriously.

It is worth noting that the term 'death drive' (which Strachey translates as 'death instinct') only appears three times in Freud's sixty-one-page text, twice in his discussion of sadism and masochism on page fifty-four, and once in a long footnote on page sixty where he attempts to clarify his terminology regarding the 'sexual instincts', the 'life instincts' and the 'death instincts'. This is perhaps somewhat surprising bearing in mind this is often regarded as Freud's seminal text on the death drive. However, the concepts of repetition and the 'tendency to zero' (Laplanche's term not Freud's, see below) are central to the paper and these link closely to the concept of the death drive.

I have already made a number of references to *Beyond the Pleasure Principle*, both in the context of the traumatic neuroses (Chap. 2) and earlier on in this chapter in relation to the pleasure principle. So rather than repeating myself I would just like to add some additional comments. The first, as I have already alluded to, concerns the concept of *repetition*, or, more precisely, what Freud describes as the 'compulsion to repeat' and which he sees as the work of the *drives*. He argues that the impulses that arise from these drives are "...*freely mobile* processes which press towards discharge."[32] He goes onto argue that the compulsion to repeat as giving "...the appearance of some daemonic force at work."[33]

[31] Richard Boothby, *Death and Desire: Psychoanalytic Theory in Lacan's Return to Freud* (Hove: Routledge, 1991), 1.

[32] Freud, 'Beyond the Pleasure Principle', 34, italics in original.

[33] *Ibid.*, 35.

And this 'daemonic force' is linked, according to Freud, to what he describes as a "universal attribute" of the drives, which is restore the living entity to an earlier state of being, which it "...has been obliged to abandon under the pressure of external disturbing forces..."[34] In essence, Freud is arguing for a drive towards an earlier, inorganic state of existence. In this sense, life is simply one long 'detour' towards death (as in reaching an inorganic, inanimate state). He acknowledges that this might seem to be a strange idea, and one which would seem to be contradicted by the fact that there appears to be an inbuilt 'survival instinct' in human beings (what Freud calls the 'ego instincts'). However, he goes onto argue that:

> The hypothesis of self-preservative instincts, such as we attribute to all living beings, stands in marked opposition to the idea that instinctual life as a whole serves to bring about death. Seen in this light, the theoretical importance of the instincts of self-preservation, of self-assertion and of mastery greatly diminishes.[35]

Another key concept in the paper is that of *binding*. Freud argues that the reaction of the psyche to the traumatic excitations is an attempt to bind the influx of energy through the process of cathexes:

> Cathectic energy is summoned from all sides to provide sufficiently high cathexes of energy in the environs of the breach. An 'anticathexis' on a grand scale is set up, for whose benefit all the other psychical systems are impoverished, so that the remaining psychical functions are extensively paralysed or reduced ... we infer that a system which is itself highly cathected is capable of taking up an additional stream of fresh inflowing energy and of converting it into quiescent cathexis, that is of binding it psychically.[36]

This process of binding energy is the basis of the pleasure principle; in other words, the lowering of excitation. What is still unclear, at least in this point of the argument, is exactly *where* this energy is coming from. At first reading it would appear that it originates in the external world,

---

[34] *Ibid.,* 36.
[35] *Ibid.,* 39.
[36] *Ibid.,* 30.

and Freud's examples of traumatic neurosis certainly include things like railway accidents and combat situations. At the same time, though, Freud is at pains to point out that traumatic neurosis does not equate with what he describes as the 'old, naive theory of shock'; rather, he argues that the traumatic neuroses are linked to the unpreparedness of the subject for the 'traumatic' event rather than the 'physicality' of the event itself. This is why Freud argues that anxiety is a *protection* against trauma, because it helps prepare the subject for the event.

Perhaps Freud's most controversial idea is that biological organisms are 'programmed' to die, or at least those that rely on sexual reproduction to propagate the species. He writes:

> If we are to take it as a truth that knows no exception that everything living dies for internal reasons—becomes inorganic once again—then we shall be compelled to say that *'the aim of all life is death'* and looking backwards, that '*inanimate things existed before living ones*'.[37]

He goes onto argue that even though more complex organisms make ever more complicated detours, their ultimate destination is still the same: death. Further on in the text, however, Freud appears to backtrack on this idea and argues instead that the self-preservative drives of the ego are libidinal and therefore should be considered as part of the sexual drives, which, according to Freud, contradict the 'drive towards death'. Such drives:

> ...are conservative in the same sense as the other instincts in that they bring back earlier states of living substance; but they are conservative to a higher degree in that they are peculiarly resistant to external influences; and they are conservative too in another sense in that they preserve life itself for a comparatively long period. They are the true life instincts.[38]

However, what Freud is actually arguing here is not that the individual organism survives but rather that sex is a way to ensure the continuity of the species through the propagation of germ cells.

---

[37] *Ibid.*, 38, italics in original.

[38] *Ibid.*, 40.

Here it should be noted that throughout the text Freud makes numerous biological and quasi-biological references, for example, the 'living substance', the 'organism, and so on. This is particularly marked in the first part of the long penultimate section of his text where he focuses on the question of biological life and death, and which revolves around a discussion of Weismann's germ theory, which in essence argues that although individual organisms may die their germ-plasma are 'immortal', in the sense they are concerned with the reproduction of the species. Freud's interest in this theory, and subsequent variations of it, lies in his search for a biological analogy that would shine light on the idea of 'natural death', that is, the innate tendency for an organism to move towards death, albeit following its own path. However, after reviewing some of the empirical literature in this field, including the work of Woodruff, Goette, and Loeb, he concluded that: "our expectation that biology would flatly contradict the recognition of death instincts has not been fulfilled."[39] In fact, the biological literature he reviewed appeared to be inconclusive on this matter.

Towards the end of the paper Freud engages in a broader discussion of the exact nature of the sexual drives and their 'beyond'. He draws upon his work on narcissism in order to show that the 'self-preservation' or ego drives are actually sexual, because in narcissism the ego takes itself as the object of the (sexual) drive. At this point Freud wonders whether there are only sexual or libidinal drives after all, and no death drive. At this point he invokes the concept of sadism but then wonders whether this is a "displaced" and "positively mystical" example of a death drive, which "...looks suspiciously as though we were trying to find a way out of a highly embarrassing situation at any price."[40] However, in a further twist of the argument he then invokes the concept of masochism as an example of a regressive drive (the complement of sadism) which *could* fit the description of the death drive because masochism "...the turning round of the instinct upon the subject's own ego, would in that case be a return to an earlier phase of the instinct's history, a regression."[41] The implication here is that primary masochism equates with the death drive.

---

[39] *Ibid.*, 49.

[40] *Ibid.*, 54.

[41] *Ibid.*, 54–55.

The Difficulties with Freud's Theory

In the final chapter in his *Life and Death in Psychoanalysis* Jean Laplanche highlights the ambiguities and contradictions in Freud's theory of the pleasure principle and its relation both to the principle of constancy and the death drive, especially as it is formulated in *Beyond the Pleasure Principle*.[42] According to Laplanche, this text "...remains the most fascinating and baffling text of the entire Freudian *corpus*." and that "Old and apparently forgotten ideas, in particular those of the *Project for a Scientific Psychology*, are taken up again and renewed."[43] He also notes that in this the question of Freud's 'biologism' comes to the fore and that a "...dialectical move "beyond" *Beyond the Pleasure Principle*, if it is to be convincing, will be possible only after the meaning of the biologism has been elucidated."[44]

Laplanche's argument in this chapter is very complex and, in some places, quite difficult to follow, but in essence he aims to demonstrate that the pleasure principle is, in fact, the principle of constancy and not, as Freud often seems to argue, a 'tendency towards zero'. In other words, the pleasure principle needs to be differentiated from the Nirvana principle, the movement of the psychical apparatus towards a null state of excitation. What Laplanche does is to highlight an underlying contradiction in Freud's concept of the pleasure principle and its relation to the principle of constancy. On the one hand, Freud seems to be trying to 'force' the principle of constancy to be a 'zero principle', in which case it becomes the Nirvana principle. On the other hand, Freud seems to be making the pleasure principle a 'modified' version of the 'zero principle' where it behaves more like the homeostatic function that the principle of constancy implies; in other words, it *regulates* energy (libido, jouissance) rather than trying to reduce it to zero. What is more puzzling, though, is why Freud ever felt the need to equate the pleasure principle/principle of constancy with the 'zero principle' in the first place; there seems to an

[42] Jean Laplanche, *Life and Death in Psychoanalysis* (Baltimore: John Hopkins University Press, 1985).

[43] *Ibid.*, 106.

[44] *Ibid.*, 106.

underlying incoherence in his argument here. Is there perhaps something in Freud's thought processes, either conscious or unconscious, that is resigned to the fact that in the end 'zero' (that is, death) always triumphs?

Laplanche argues that for Freud the 'tendency towards zero' (the Nirvana principle) is the radical form of the pleasure principle. This not only clearly contradicts, as Laplanche notes, the 'masochistic search for unpleasure', but perhaps more importantly, the increase in tension (excitation) brought about by trauma. In other words, if the death drive is the tendency towards zero, it cannot also be attributed to trauma, that is, drive-jouissance. The key point here is that constancy (homeostasis) does not in itself imply a 'zero state' of excitation. In principle it could be maintained at a very high level, as long as it remained constant. The problem that Laplanche is highlighting is that it is unclear in Freud's work, especially in *Beyond the Pleasure Principle*, whether in fact he (Freud) thinks that pleasure principle equates with the principle of constancy which in turn equates with the 'tendency towards zero'. If this is the case then the pleasure principle, as the principle of constancy, effectively becomes the death drive.

Laplanche points out that for Freud the 'zero principle' is identified with free energy, the primary process, and the pleasure principle. And pleasure is defined as the sensation of discharge (of energy). On this basis, the principle of constancy becomes linked to *bound* energy and the *secondary* process, whereas the pleasure principle is linked free (unbound) energy and the primary process. However, as Laplanche goes on to argue, in *Beyond the Pleasure Principle* Freud 'modifies' the notion of the pleasure principle:

> The displacement of the term "pleasure principle" should not mislead us: the pleasure principle, insofar as, throughout the text, it is posited as being of a piece with its "modification" as the reality principle, is henceforth situated on the side of constancy. It is "its most radical form" or its "*beyond*" which, as the Nirvana principle, reasserts the priority of the tendency towards absolute zero of the "death drive."[45]

[45] *Ibid.*, 117, italics in original.

This goes a long way to explaining Freud's apparently surprising statement at the end of *Beyond the Pleasure Principle* that the pleasure principle is in the service of the death drive. In its most 'radical' form the pleasure principle *is* the death drive. On this basis too, libido, as an excess of excitation, is *opposed* to the death drive, insofar as the death drive 'aims at zero'. It also begs the question as to why Freud felt the need to describe the death drive as being 'beyond' the pleasure principle in the first place, when clearly it is not. Or, rather, it is only 'beyond' insofar as the pleasure principle is 'modified' to become the principle of constancy.

One question that remains unanswered, however, in Laplanche's approach to the pleasure principle and its relation to the death drive is the role of *language* and the Symbolic register in general in regulating libido and therefore trauma. In his later text, *New Foundations for Psychoanalysis,* he argues that language, and specifically verbal language, is *secondary* in Freud's work. By this he does not mean that language is of no importance to Freud, but, rather, that language is derived from more fundamental and non-linguistic processes. According to Laplanche, language is secondary in *historical* terms, that is, in terms of history of the subject, and that there exists a pre-verbal stage; it is also secondary in *topographical* terms because, argues Laplanche, for Freud consciousness is primarily a perceptual consciousness, which means language, in the form of word presentations, follow from perception; and finally, language is secondary in *economic* terms, by which Laplanche means it is "...governed by a mode of association and circulation which involves barriers and dams."[46] What Laplanche appears to be getting at here is language itself has to be regulated in order to prevent an endless circulation of meaning.

Laplanche does, however, acknowledge the importance of the *signifier*, although he argues against Lacan's privileging of it. Instead, he makes a distinction between a signifier *of*, that is, giving meaning, and a signifier *to*, which refers to the *effect* a signifier can have without necessarily conveying meaning: "A signifier has a discernible significance, and a signifying or significant power; we know that *there is 'a signifying'* somewhere,

[46] *Ibid.*, 43.

but there is not necessarily any explicit signified."[47] He refers to the idea of the signifier as 'designified', which forms the basis for his theory of the 'enigmatic signifier' which will play a key role in his approach to *Nachträglichkeit* and the idea of childhood seduction.

However, Laplanche's approach to the pleasure principle does play down the importance of language. At the same time, he acknowledges the influence of Fechner and psychophysics in Freud's theory of the pleasure principle and this, I argue, creates a problem. As it stands, that is, bereft of the dimension of language, Freud's (and, by extension, Laplanche's) theory of the pleasure principle remains 'trapped', so to speak, within the discourse of *energetics*, by which I mean the idea that the pleasure principle/principle of constancy is a 'mechanism' for regulating free-flowing energy within the psychical apparatus. It was this focus on energy and its regulation that provided the basis for Fechner's theory of psychophysics; and, perhaps more problematically for contemporary psychoanalysis, provides one of the theoretical foundations for modern day attempts to 'combine' psychoanalysis and neuroscience.[48]

The main problem here, in my view, is not so much Freud's use of the language of psychophysics per se, which as both Hawkins and Ellenberger point out was by no means a 'reductionist' theory of the psyche; but rather, by default it effectively 'sidelines' the importance of language; or, referring back to Laplanche's argument, makes language 'secondary'. In other words, as they stand, Freud's theories of the pleasure principle, the principle of constancy and the death drive are in danger of 'collapsing' into some form of (quasi) neurobiologism. It is for this reason, I argue, that Lacan's approach to the pleasure principle is so critical, because it provides an escape route from such dangers.

---

[47] *Ibid.*, 45, italics in original.

[48] See, for example, Thomas Rabeyron's paper on Freud's 'energetics' theory and its relation to modern neuroscience: Thomas Rabeyron, 'Psychoanalytic Psychotherapies and the Free Energy Principle', *Frontiers in Human Neuroscience*, 16 (2022). The 'modernisation' of Fechner's and James' work is discussed by Hawkins in the paper already cited.

Lacan, the Pleasure Principle and the Machine of Language

Lacan's position with regards to the pleasure principle is inextricably tied up with his approach to language and the nature of the Symbolic register, and this becomes especially clear in lessons three to seven of his second seminar, and also in lesson twenty-three.[49] One of the key themes in the seminar is the idea of the *machine* and how this relates to language. In many ways this seems to prefigure Lacan's argument in *Seminar XI* regarding Lacan's use of the Aristotelian concept of the *automaton* and its relation to the Symbolic register. However, in *Seminar II* the emphasis is more on the idea of the self-regulating machine and how this relates to ideas concerning energy, homeostasis and entropy, which, argues Lacan, are key concepts in modern biology and physics, and are also relevant to discussions regarding the pleasure principle and the principle of constancy.

In lesson five of *Seminar II* Lacan discusses the idea of an internal organisation in the psyche "…which up to a certain point tends to oppose the free and unlimited passage of forces and discharges of energy…".[50] This internal organisation includes the operation of homeostasis, "…which absorbs, moderates the irruption of quantities of energy *coming from the external world*."[51] This is essentially following Freud's argument in *Beyond the Pleasure Principle*, where the pleasure principle regulates the excitations emanating from the external world. It is interesting to note that Lacan, in this passage, is also arguing that the excitations are *external*.

The aim of homeostasis is to restore a state of equilibrium in the psychical apparatus. However, Lacan goes on to note that Freud had realised that there is something that does not satisfy the pleasure principle, which manifests itself as the compulsion to repeat. Lacan also notes that

[49] Jacques Lacan, *The Seminar of Jacques Lacan. Book II: The Ego in Freud's Theory and in the Technique of Psychoanalysis 1954–1955* (Cambridge: Cambridge University Press, 1988). (Hereafter *Seminar II*)

[50] *Ibid.*, 60.

[51] *Ibid.*, 60, my italics.

repetition in dreams in cases of traumatic neuroses contravene the rule of the pleasure principle, that is, wish fulfilment. Later on in the Seminar (in lesson seven) he argues that:

> From the beginning of Freud's work to the end, the pleasure principle is explained in the following way—when faced with a stimulus encroaching on the living apparatus, the nervous system is as it were the indispensable delegate of the homeostat, of the indispensable regulator, thanks to which the living being survives, and to which corresponds a tendency to lower the excitation to a minimum. *To a minimum*, what does that mean? There is an ambiguity here, which puts analytic authors under some difficulty.[52]

This ambiguity, according to Lacan, revolves around the fact that 'minimum', from a biological perspective, can mean either to reach a certain point of equilibrium, or an absolute minimum, that is, death. It also highlights a certain tension and ambiguity in Freud's writings about the pleasure principle and may well be linked to his (over) reliance on biological models. This is the idea, as noted above by Lacan, that the concept of the regulation of excitation can either mean that the excitation is kept at a particular level at some point above zero, or it can mean a reduction to zero. As I noted earlier, this is something that Laplanche takes up in his discussion of the death drive.

What's perhaps even more interesting, however, is that Lacan is attempting to address the relation of the biological organism to the *machine* and the idea of the *mechanism*. For example, in lesson three he states:

> Thus, when it comes down to it, we always try to explain the living organism in terms of mechanism. The first question which we analysts must answer, and which can perhaps help us get away from the controversy which exists between vitalism and mechanism, is the following—why are we led to think of life in terms of mechanism?[53]

[52] *Ibid.*, 80, italics in original.

[53] *Ibid.*, 31.

Lacan goes onto to point out that the concept of the *mechanism* in philosophy had changed quite considerably since its introduction in the eighteenth century, especially since the advent of the steam engine, where the emphasis shifted to the idea of regulated energy (through the use of the self-regulator valve), and even more so with the advent of cybernetics in the mid-twentieth century. Cybernetics is especially important here because it allows Lacan to make a direct connection between language and the machine (mechanism) and which he discusses at some length in lesson twenty-three of *Seminar II*.[54] It is also an opportunity for Lacan to discuss his ideas regarding the 'exact sciences' (physics, astronomy, etc) and their relation to the Real. Lacan argues that the exact sciences were born out of the realisation that certain human actions, for example rites, dances and magical invocations, had very little influence on the natural order of things: "From the moment man thinks that the great clock of nature turns all by itself, and continues to mark the hour even when he isn't there, the order of science is born."[55]

And one of the key aspects of modern science, according to Lacan, is that it 'reduces' the Real to a small number of symbols (signifiers). It is important to note that in this seminar Lacan refers to the Real as "...something one always finds in the same place, whether or not one has been there."[56] In other words, the Real is that which exists independently of human thought or perception, for example (which is the one Lacan uses) the stars in the sky. And sticking with this example, celestial bodies (stars, planets, and so on) domain can be 'reduced' to a set of mathematical equations that plot their orbits, evolution and eventual decay. Such equations can be manipulated mathematically, for example using the probability calculus, which Lacan argues appears in its first truly scientific form in Pascal's treatise on the arithmetic triangle, and which, according to Lacan, constitutes the first machine.[57] Lacan uses the model of such a

[54] Which is a presentation of the final lecture in a special series on the theme of 'Psychoanalysis and the human sciences' organised by the *Société Française de Psychanalyse* and delivered by Lacan on 22 June 1955.

[55] *Ibid.*, 298.

[56] *Ibid.*, 297.

[57] It appears, though not stated explicitly in the text, that Lacan may here be conflating Pascal's arithmetic *triangle* with his arithmetic *machine* (the 'Pascaline Calculator') which is generally regarded as the world's first genuine arithmetical calculator.

machine to emphasise the idea of the order of symbols being characterised by presence and absence. Somewhat surprisingly, perhaps, he uses the example of a gambler to illustrate this idea:

> What Pascal develops with the arithmetic triangle, the first machine, has a claim on the attention of the scientific world, in that it enables one to determine immediately what a gambler has the right to expect at any given moment when the succession of turns which makes up a game is interrupted. A succession of turns is the simplest form one can give to the idea of the encounter … What's at issue is the place, what does or doesn't come to fill it…[58]

In symbolic (and machine) terms, absence and presence can be represented in *binary code*, that is, as a series of 0 s and 1 s. This, argues Lacan, is the key to the development of cybernetics along with the introduction of what he calls the 'cybernetised doors', by which he appears to be referring to the electronic switches that form the basis of cybernetic and computer circuits:

> Once the door (switch) is open, it closes. When it is closed, it opens … Thanks to the electrical circuit, and to the induction circuit connected on to it, that is to say what is called feedback, it's sufficient for the door to close for it to be returned by an electro-magnet to an open state and that is its closure again, and its opening again. In that way what is called an oscillation is produced.[59]

It is important to note that Lacan was making these arguments on the cusp of the computer age and so perhaps was not able to fully appreciate the strength of his own models and analogies. In hindsight, perhaps, it is much clearer that he was prefiguring the advent of computers and the machine languages that program them (binary and hexadecimal codes). This is something that John Johnston discusses in some depth in his study

[58] *Ibid.*, 299.

[59] *Ibid.*, 302.

of cybernetics, artificial intelligence (AI) and artificial life (ALife).[60] He points out that *Seminar II* was held in the wake of the last Macy Conference, the tenth in a series of conferences held in New York City from 1946 to 1953, and which brought together mathematicians, scientists, engineers, psychiatrists, anthropologists and social scientists in order to discuss a range of topics revolving around the theme of 'feedback mechanisms and circular causal systems in biology and the social sciences'. During this period, cybernetics was in its ascendence, and the conferences themselves were organised by one of the leading researchers in the field, Norbert Wiener. Johnston goes on to note that although it is not clear how much Lacan would have known about the Macy Conferences, he certainly knew about much of the research that was being conducted in the field of cybernetics, and, furthermore, would have discussed such matters with Roman Jakobson (a major influence on Lacan) who taught at MIT where both Wiener and Claude Shannon, another key figure in the cybernetics world, were professors. In other words, Lacan's ideas on language and cybernetics would undoubtedly have been informed by the latest thinking in this area, whilst at the same time he would have been unable to fully appreciate what was to follow in the broader field of computer science and AI.

Johnston argues that:

> Lacan's machines are really information machines, simple ones at that, since all they do is count, store, and integrate codings of binary numbers (1s and 0s). Yet these basic operations underlie all that a modern digital computer does. Since the computer, or rather its conceptual forerunner, Alan Turing's universal machine of 1936, is the most important technological invention between Freud and Lacan, Lacan's rewriting of Freud should be understood as an attempt to redefine the psychic apparatus according to contemporary conditions of mediality.[61]

---

[60] John Johnston, *The Allure of Machinic Life: Cybernetics, Artificial Life and the New AI* (Cambridge, Massachusetts: MIT Press, 2008).

[61] *Ibid.*, 81–82.

Here Johnston is drawing on the work of media theorist Friedrich Kittler who argued that Lacan was essentially rewriting Freud's theory of the psychical apparatus in the light of contemporary media and information theory:

> Freud's materialism reasoned only as far as the information machines of his era-no more, no less. Rather than continuing to dream of the Spirit as origin, he described a "psychic apparatus" (Freud's wonderful word choice) that implemented all available transmission and storage media, in other words, an apparatus just short of the technical medium of universal-calculation, or the computer.[62]

Lacan, on the other hand, could draw on the work of the (nascent) computer and information scientists, including Wiener and Shannon, and one of the key findings here that Lacan utilises in his theory of language is the idea of *negative entropy.* Interestingly, the concept of entropy itself, that is, the tendency of energy systems to move towards an irreversible state of disorder or randomness, would have been known to Freud and yet the term only appears once in the whole of *The Standard Edition.*[63] This seems rather peculiar because the concept would appear to epitomise the idea of a movement from the organic to the inorganic, that is, a central tenet of Freud's arguments in *Beyond the Pleasure Principle.* In information theory, Claude Shannon utilised the ideas of Ludwig Boltzmann (who developed the formula for computing entropy in a thermodynamic system) in order to address the problem of uncertainty in the transmission of messages:

> For Shannon, the uncertainty of a message stems from the freedom of choice in the selection of a particular message (or set of symbols constituting a message). The greater the number of possible messages, the greater the uncertainty and hence the greater the information value of a single selected message or symbol.[64]

---

[62] Friedrich A. Kittler, 'The World of the Symbolic, A World of the Machine', in *Literature, Media, Information Systems*, ed. by John Johnston (London: Taylor & Francis Group, 1997), p. 134.

[63] Sigmund Freud, 'From the History of an Infantile Neurosis', in *The Standard Edition of the Complete Psychological Works of Sigmund Freud* (London: Hogarth Press, 1918), XVII, 116.

[64] Johnston, *The Allure of Machinic Life*, 28.

Lacan draws on the arguments of Norbert Weiner[65] and the idea that information measures a *gain in certainty* in a message system, which is another way of saying that information counters entropy:

> The phenomena of energy and of nature always tend in the direction of an equalisation of levels of difference ('the reduction to zero'). In the order of the message and of the calculation of chances, to the extent that the information increases, the difference in levels becomes more differentiated.[66]

In other words, any system of circulating symbols tends towards organisation and order, rather than disorder and randomness. And, according to Lacan, this is precisely the characteristic of the Symbolic register itself. However, at this point it is important to note, as does Johnston in his discussion of the Seminar, that Lacan never identifies the Symbolic with language:

> ...rather, he understands the symbolic order as operating within or by means of language, in and by means of specific circuits of discourse in which signs of recognition or exchange are passed or not passed. Importantly, the operations of the symbolic order are never confused with or reduced to the operations of language.[67]

Although this might at first sight appear to be a rather surprising assertion, a closer examination reveals that what Johnston is actually arguing, and this is clear from Lacan's cybernetics lecture, is that by 'language' he is referring to *natural* language, not language per se. As Johnston points out, "...it was Lacan's familiarity with finite-state automata that enabled him to understand that simple information machines were not unlike simple restricted languages with a limited set of functions..."[68] This is

[65] Although he doesn't directly cite Weiner at this point.

[66] Lacan, *Seminar II*, 305.

[67] Johnston, *The Allure of Machinic Life*, 88.

[68] *Ibid.*, 88. By 'finite-state automata' Johnston is referring to the idea, originally formulated by Alan Turing in 1936, that if a problem can be expressed as an algorithm (a precise set of instructions for arriving at a specified solution) then it can be computed mechanically, that is, by a machine. This then gave rise to the question as to whether such a machine would ever arrive at a finite answer. Without going into the technical details Turing's answer was yes, the machine would halt with a finite answer, hence the term 'finite-state automata'. Furthermore, this would form one of the key conceptual and technological building blocks of modern computing.

also what leads Lacan to argue that in any language system *syntax* takes priority over *semantics*:

> In order for language to come into being, insignificant little things such as spelling and syntax have to be introduced … In other words, within this perspective, syntax exists before semantics. Cybernetics is a science of syntax, and it is in a good position to help us perceive that the exact sciences do nothing other than tie the real to a syntax.[69]

What Lacan is getting at here is the idea that the Symbolic register is based on an encoding of the Real, using binary logic (1 s and 0 s), in a machine-like configuration not unlike that of modern computer systems. Presumably (although he does not state this explicitly in the Seminar), more complex, natural languages can be developed on the basis of this binary foundation in the same way complex computer programs can be built on computer machine code. At this point, of course, it could be argued that Lacan is simply substituting a cybernetic/computer science model for Freud's psychophysical one. In fact, a 'cybernetic' theory of language raises an important question regarding the relationship between Freud's energetics and Lacan's use of cybernetics, game and information theory. Concepts such as information flow, entropy and negative entropy are essentially derived from physics and treat networks of information, broadly speaking, in the same way as networks of energy. In other words, cybernetics and information theory starts to look like a latter-day version of nineteenth century energetics and psychophysics. Although, as I argue at the end of this chapter, things are not that simple, it is true to say that many of these ideas have now been updated and are currently being applied (erroneously I would argue) in various attempts to 'fuse' psychoanalysis with neuroscience.[70]

---

[69] Lacan, *Seminar II*, 305.

[70] For a useful rebuttal of such arguments see Eric Laurent, *Lost in Cognition: Psychoanalysis and the Cognitive Sciences* (London: Karnac, 2014) and Yves Vanderveken, "The Unconscious and the Brain: Nothing in Common," *The Lacanian Review*, no. 09 (2020): 198–213.

The Purloined Lacan and the Cybernetic Unconscious

Many of the ideas that I have explored above relating to cybernetics and language have also been explored in some depth by Lydia Liu in her book *The Freudian Robot*, and especially in the chapter entitled 'The Cybernetic Unconscious'.[71] Liu's arguments are important, in my view, because (like Johnston's, which I discussed earlier) they raise some important questions regarding Lacan's theory of language and especially how it has been 'translated' (both literally and metaphorically) by the Anglo-American academy. Like Johnston, Liu is particularly interested in Lacan's arguments in *Seminar II* relating to language and cybernetics. Unlike him, however, her interest is more on the broader implications regarding different 'readings' of Lacan and her rather interesting perspective on how 'French Theory' was accommodated by the North American academic community and how this relates to the question of the cybernetic unconscious of the post-war Euro-(North) American world order.

One of her key arguments is that much of so-called 'French Theory' "...was already a translation of American theory before it landed in America to be reinvented as French theory."[72] This matters, according to Liu, because what had been 'translated' from the American theory into French theory (in France) in the early 1950s were critical ideas relating to game theory, language and cybernetics. By the time it had been 'retranslated' and sent back to the universities of North America (and various other Anglophone countries) from the 1970s onwards, particularly in the guise of poststructuralism, many of the crucial elements of the original translation had been lost. Liu cites one example of the French mathematicians' reception of John von Neumann and Oskar Morgenstern's game theory applied to economics and nuclear warfare. She points out that the French term *jeu* can mean either 'game' or 'play' in English. The French mathematicians opted for the former but in its journey back to North America the emphasis shifted to the latter meaning, that is, 'play'. This

[71] Lydia H. Liu, *The Freudian Robot: Digital Media and the Future of the Unconscious* (Chicago: The University of Chicago Press, 2010).

[72] *Ibid.*, 153.

matters, according to Liu, because the adoption of the word 'play' instead of 'game' served to obscure the more sinister connotations of game theory, that is, as a way to help the USA win both economic and military wars.

Crucially, what Liu is arguing is that what gets 'lost in translation' is a whole theory of language and, consequently, a whole theory of the unconscious; rather than a theory based on cybernetics, information theory, game theory and so on, what becomes adopted in North American (and other) academies is a completely different understanding of language from the one Lacan was developing in *Seminar II*. And one of the main reasons for this is that the mid-1950s also saw the emergence of structuralism, and, of particular importance to Lacan's future teaching, the rise of structural linguistics, which revolved around the ideas of Saussure, Jakobson and others. The influence of Saussure's ideas in particular feature prominently in many Lacanian texts, and especially the more introductory ones.[73] However, according to Liu, this is a mistake. She points to the fact that a key part of Lacan's reading of Saussure was to invert his (Saussure's) model of the sign and to place the signified *under* the signifier. And part of the reason for this inversion was to emphasise the priority of the signifier over the signified. She makes reference to a passage from lesson seven of *Seminar II*, where Lacan is discussing Claude Shannon's work at Bell Labs (although as Liu points out he omits to name Shannon). The focus here is on Shannon's idea that in order to economise on its wiring of telecommunications, messages are encoded before transmission and decoded on receipt. The *meaning* of such messages becomes irrelevant. According to Liu "…Shannon would have been in complete agreement with Lacan about the quantification of communication, the need to economize, the irrelevance of sense to a message…"[74]

She goes onto to argue that:

[73] See for example Joël Dor's *Introduction to the Reading of Lacan: The Unconscious Is Structured Like a Language* (New York: The Other Press, 1998), and Bruce Fink's *The Lacanian Subject* Bruce Fink, *The Lacanian Subject: Between Language and Jouissance* (Princeton: Princeton University Press, 1995).

[74] Liu, *The Freudian Robot,* 189.

> This provides a clear explanation as to why Lacan decided to reverse the position of signifier and signified in Saussure's diagram, and it also outlines the general direction in which Lacan conceptualizes the unconscious in relation to the symbolic order. The material language, which is the instrument of speech, is no longer the same as the Saussurian language. Rather, it operates in the manner of a telephone exchange system or a cybernetic machine that runs automatically regardless of what happens to pass down its wires.[75]

In contrast, the 'Saussurian Lacan' places the emphasis on *meaning*, on the *signified*, and not enough on the signifier itself; what Lacan in other texts will refer to as 'the letter' or 'the unary trait'. Liu makes reference to Lacan's attempt to rectify this over-emphasis on the signified: "In his 1971 seminar, he tried to rectify that misunderstanding by claiming that 'it is not for nothing that I have written *the instance of the letter in the unconscious.* I have never said *the instance of the signified*'."[76] This might sound rather surprising, bearing in mind that most Lacanian texts place a great deal of emphasis on the signifier. However, I would argue that such an emphasis is taking place *within the framework of the signified*; in other words, although the focus is on the signifier, the emphasis is on what this *means*. The problem here, I would argue, is that this fails to recognise the 'machine-like' nature of the operation of the signifier (and of language itself) which Lacan is trying to convey throughout *Seminar II*.

But how does this relate to the idea of the *unconscious*, and especially to what Liu refers to as the 'cybernetic unconscious'? In lesson 22 of *Seminar II* Lacan becomes embroiled in a difficult exchange with his audience, many of whom seem to be perplexed by Lacan's arguments regarding numbers and language. At one point Lacan states:

> When one illustrates the phenomenon of language with something as formally purified as mathematical symbols—and that is one of the reasons for putting cybernetics on the agenda—when one gives a mathematical

[75] *Ibid.*, 189.

[76] *Ibid.*, 95, italics in original.

> notation of the *verbum*, one demonstrates in the simplest possible way that language exists completely independently of us. Numbers have properties which are absolute. They are, whether we're here or not … All this can circulate in all manner of ways in the universal machine, which is more universal than anything you could imagine. One can imagine an indefinite number of levels, where all this turns around and circulates. The world of signs functions, and it has no signification whatsoever.[77]

Here Lacan is reiterating his idea that the basis of language is a binary code, which represents presence and absence. Further on Lacan argues that:

> …the circulation of binary signs in a machine enables us, if we give it the right programme, to discover a previously unpublished prime number. The prime number circulating in the machine has got nothing to do with thought.[78]

Liu, in her reading of this passage, argues that this shows that it is the unconscious, not the speaking subject, that thinks and "…plays the game of chances according to given combinatory rules".[79] In this sense, the unconscious is the endless circuit of signifiers (1 s and 0 s, pluses and minuses) which lies beyond the conscious thought of individual subjects. Furthermore, and this is especially pertinent to my discussion in the next chapter, the idea of such an endless circuit of signifiers resonates very closely with Lacan's use of the Aristotelian concept of *automaton*.

The Death Drive and the Symbolic Register

The essence of Freud's theory of the pleasure principle, in spite of all the problems it presents, is that it regulates the free-flow of energy in the psychical apparatus; or, in Lacanian terms, it regulates the jouissance of

---

[77] Lacan, *Seminar II*, 284.

[78] *Ibid.*, 286.

[79] Liu, *The Freudian Robot*, 191.

the drive. Using Lacan's 'cybernetic model' of the structure and circulation of language it can be seen that such a system can be regarded as 'self-regulating' and is constantly moving to a state of homeostasis and order, as opposed to a state of entropy and disorder. At this point it should be reiterated that by 'language' we are not talking about *natural* language but a more 'basic' system of binary coding. However, as Lacan points out, there is something else present in the system that disrupts such orderliness, and this something else is the death drive:

> In effect, according to the hypothesis of the pleasure principle, the entire system should always return to its starting-point, should always act in a homeostatic way ... How is it that there is something which, from whatever end we approach it, does not fit into the movement, into the framework of the pleasure principle? ... This is precisely why he (Freud) was led straight to the function of the death instinct [sic].[80]

But how exactly does Lacan conceptualise this death drive, this 'something that doesn't fit'? Right at the end of the last lesson of *Seminar II*, where he has been discussing the ego in relation to the Imaginary, Lacan states:

> The symbolic order is rejected by the libidinal order, which includes the whole of the domain of the imaginary, including the structure of the ego. And the death instinct [drive] is only the mask of symbolic order, in so far—this is what Freud writes—as it is dumb, that is to say in so far as it hasn't been realised ... The symbolic order is simultaneously non-being and insisting to be, that is what Freud has in mind when he talks about the death instinct as being what is most fundamental—a symbolic order in travail, in the process of coming, insisting on being realised.[81]

In other words, Lacan is making the somewhat remarkable claim that the death drive is related to the Symbolic register itself; more precisely, it is

[80] Lacan, *Seminar II*, 66.
[81] *Ibid.*, 326.

the Symbolic register in the process of becoming. This seems a long way from Freud's concept of the death drive as a 'reduction to zero' but makes more sense if we consider Lacan's argument in *Seminar VII* that the death drive should not be viewed in terms of a theory of energetics but, rather, as a theory of the signifier and language. In order to explain this assertion he makes what appears to be a rather unusual excursion into Sade's *Juliette* where he (Sade) discourses on the System of Pope Pius VI. According to Lacan:

> Sade lays out for our benefit the theory that it is through crime that man collaborates in the new creations of nature. The idea is that the pure force of nature is obstructed by its own forms, that because the three realms present fixed forms they bind nature to a limited cycle … As a result, the deepest concern that can be imputed to this psychic subject that is Nature is that of wanting to wipe the slate clean, so that it may begin its task once more, set out again with a new burst of energy.[82]

In other words, destruction is the catalyst of renewal and creation. As Lacan notes, although Sade's language is more poetic than scientific, he is nevertheless making an important point that any evolutionist would recognise. More crucially for Lacan's argument regarding the death drive, however, is that it is not situated on the side of some form of 'annihilation principle', which "…concerns a relationship to a fundamental law which might be identified with that which energetics theorizes as the tendency to return to a state, if not of absolute rest, then at least of universal equilibrium." Rather, the death drive "…is to be situated in the historical domain: it is articulated at a level that can only be defined as a function of the signifying chain…"[83]

[82] Jacques Lacan, *The Ethics of Psychoanalysis 1959–1960 The Seminar of Jacques Lacan Book VII* (London: Routledge, 1992), 210. (Hereafter *Seminar VII*)

[83] *Ibid.*, 211.

Conclusion: From Psychophysics to Cybernetics (Via French Theory)

I would like to end this chapter by discussing in a little more detail the relationship between Lacan's teachings and 'French Theory', particularly in the light of Lydia Liu's claim that such a theory had led to a misunderstanding of his work.

In his book *Why there is no Poststructuralism in France,* Johannes Angermuller argues that poststructuralism (which is his term for Liu's 'French Theory') was essentially an invention of the North American academy in the 1970s.[84] More specifically, it was an invention of certain English Literature departments within the academy and before long also found its way into cultural studies' departments. As the title of his book suggests, in France the term 'poststructuralism' has hardly ever been recognised, and none of the so-called 'poststructuralist' thinkers (Derrida, Foucault, Lacan, and so on) would ever have recognised this label during their own lifetime. But this is not the end of the story. For not only was the idea of poststructuralism/French Theory invented in North America but it was soon 'exported' back to Europe. Interestingly, Angermuller includes thinkers such as Slavoj Žižek and Alain Badiou amongst these European 'poststructuralists', which is somewhat ironic bearing in mind that Žižek in particular would be the first to renounce such a label. Angermuller's argument certainly seems to give more credence to Liu's thesis regarding the fate of Lacan's 'cybernetic' theory of language; namely that it became 'lost in translation' during its criss-crossing of the Atlantic. However, there seem to be some serious difficulties is sustaining the idea that its purely the fault of 'French Theory' (or simply 'Theory' as Angermuller puts it) that such a 'cybernetic' reading of Lacan has become 'lost'. And the biggest difficulty of all, I would argue, is that after *Seminar II* Lacan himself seems to 'lose' the idea; there are very few references to cybernetics in his subsequent works, whereas there are, of course, a great deal of references to the operation of the signifier, which features heavily in much structuralist and poststructuralist thought.

---

[84] Johannes Angermuller, *Why There Is No Poststructuralism in France The Making of an Intellectual Generation* (London: Bloomsbury Academic, 2015).

However, this hardly makes the case for a 'Saussurian' or (post)structuralist Lacan. After all, the signifier is not an invention of structural linguistics. And as Liu is at pains to point out, one of the first things Lacan did with Saussure's theory of the sign was to invert it and place the signifier above the signified. Furthermore, and as Liu also notes, it was none other than Jacques Derrida, the 'darling' of French Theory, who in the first chapter of *Of Grammatology* made some very interesting references to cybernetics in relation to the field of writing:

> And, finally, whether it has essential limits or not, the entire field covered by the cybernetic *program* will be the field of writing. If the theory of cybernetics is by itself to oust any metaphysical concepts-including the concepts of soul, of life, of value, of choice, of memory-which until recently served to separate the machine from man, it must conserve the notion of writing, trace, grammè [written mark], or grapheme, until its own historico-metaphysical character is also exposed.[85]

Liu points out that Derrida was writing this at a time when molecular biology and its language of 'coding' and 'decoding' was replacing the older biological discourse of 'organs' and 'organisms', which is something Derrida himself references in his text. The key point here is that the influence of cybernetics and information theory was reaching into disciplines which, up until that point (the early to mid-1960s) would not have seen them as relevant. Perhaps it could be argued that in many ways Lacan was ahead of the game, because he had recognised already in the early 1950s that Freudian psychophysics could be 'rewritten' in the language of cybernetics.

As for the fact that Lacan did not continue to reference cybernetics in his teaching after *Seminar II*, the key point here is that he did not have to. By using the model of cybernetics he had already established (in *Seminar II*) that the Symbolic register (and therefore the unconscious) is structured and operates as an automatous and self-regulating machine based

[85] Jacques Derrida, *Of Grammatology*, Corrected Edition (Baltimore: The Johns Hopkins University Press, 1997), 9, italics in original.

on discrete 'bits' of information (individual signifiers). So it is no surprise, for instance, that in *Seminar XI* he will equate Aristotle's idea of the *automaton* with the Symbolic register. And the idea of the endless repetition of the drive and the relationship between jouissance and language can all be conceptualised within a cybernetic framework. In other words, there is nothing in Lacan's later work that undermines his teachings in *Seminar II* regarding the pivotal role of cybernetics in relation to the pleasure principle, language and the drive.

However, this does *not* mean that Lacan's theories should be reinterpreted within the framework of computer science; for example, the mind as an information processing machine (the model of cognitive psychology), anymore than his work should be reinterpreted within the framework of neurobiology. Clearly, it might be tempting to argue that by using the language of cybernetics and information theory, Lacan is simply 'updating' Freud's 'biologism' into a new discourse, which is something I alluded to earlier. However, it is important to recognise that such a 'biologism' is not simply a precursor to modern neurobiology; as I noted in my discussion of psychophysics, for theorists such as Fechner psychophysics had very little to do with a crude and reductive materialism. Likewise, I would argue that with Lacan he is not arguing that the human psyche is 'reducible' to a set of neural networks that are structured like a computer. Rather, he is proposing a theory of language based on the automatous and repetitive nature of the signifier.

However, perhaps there is a broader issue at stake here. In my view it is not a question of one 'reading' of Lacan 'versus' another; for example, a 'cybernetic reading' versus a 'Saussurian reading'. Rather, it is a question of taking a more critical and sceptical stance regarding *any* 'reading'. The thrust of Liu's argument is that because so many Lacanian academics and analysts over the years have adopted a 'Saussurian' or 'poststructuralist' reading of Lacan they have failed to recognise how much his teachings in the early to mid-1950s were influenced by information theory and cybernetics. This has essentially become 'lost in translation'. The danger here, though, is to go to the other extreme and opt for a 'cybernetic' reading of Lacan which would be to the detriment of much of his other teaching. Liu is correct when she argues that Lacan was no 'Saussurian' and that he adapted Saussure's theory for his own ends. But, likewise, he did this with many other theories including Hegel's, Lévi-Strauss', Jakobson's, and, it could be argued, with Freud's himself. In other words, Lacan did not appear to be especially (ideologically or transferentially) 'tied' to any specific theory or theorist; rather, he utilised whichever aspect of a particular theory that suited his own needs at the time.

But going back to my earlier claim that Lacan, through his use of cybernetic and information theory, was developing a theory of the signifier, such a theory of the signifier is closely linked to a theory of the human subject, and it is here that the Lacanian idea of an 'inaugural trauma' enters the picture. But this is not *any* subject; rather, and this is the focus of the following chapter, according to Lacan this is the subject of modern, mathematically based science. Furthermore, it is *this* subject that makes psychoanalysis possible in the first place and it is to this subject that we must now turn.

4

An Inaugural Trauma?

Introduction

> Human beings are living creatures capable of speech and, as such, have been exiled from the animal kingdom regulated by the logic of the natural satisfaction of needs. Lacan describes as "real jouissance" such unmediated satisfaction as is sought by the animal who pounces on its prey out of hunger or follows the rhythms of its mating instinct. But however far back one goes in the life of a human being, one cannot find any trace of access to that real jouissance. Language has transformed us into beings subject to a logic that is other than biological or natural logic.[1]

As the above quote from Lucie Cantin suggests, for Lacanians the human subject is brought into being or 'inaugurated' by a trauma; and this is the trauma of the human being's entry into language. In this chapter I will explore this process of 'inauguration' in some detail and the focal point of my discussion will be Lacan's *Science and Truth*, which has been

[1] Lucie Cantin, 'The Trauma of Language', in *After Lacan: Clinical Practice and the Subject of the Unconscious*, ed. by Robert Hughes and Kareen Malone (Albany: State University of New York Press, 2002), 35.

© The Author(s), under exclusive license to Springer Nature Switzerland AG 2025

L. Chapman, *Traumatic Neurosis Revisited*, The Palgrave Lacan Series,
https://doi.org/10.1007/978-3-031-89158-8_4

published as a separate text within the *Écrits*,[2] but also forms the basis of the first lesson of Lacan's *Seminar XIII*.[3] In the course of my discussion I will also be examining Lacan's ideas relating to trauma, cause and the Real in *Seminar XI* and Miller's discussion of the concept of 'suture' in his paper of the same title. The crux of my argument in this chapter is that the subject of language is also, and somewhat paradoxically, the subject of the Real, and in this latter sense it can be argued that the subject *is* trauma. However, before proceeding with my main discussion I would like to say a few words regarding my rationale for focusing on Lacan's *Science and Truth*.

As I've just indicated, *Science and Truth* was originally the first lesson in Lacan's seminar of 1965–1966 *The Object of Psychoanalysis*. The lesson itself was presented on 1 December 1965. The text of the lesson was then published in the first issue of *Cahiers Pour l'Analyse* in January 1966. I highlight these dates because they are over twelve years after Lacan presented his paper *The Function and Field of Speech and Language in Psychoanalysis* in Rome in September 1953 (often referred to as 'The Rome Discourse'), which was subsequently published in the *Écrits*.[4] It could perhaps be argued that the Rome Discourse is very much an 'inaugural' text in its own right with regards to Lacan's teaching, and although his ideas evolved, often in quite radical ways, over the next twenty years or so, many of the key Lacanian concepts are already present in this text. And perhaps the most important of these concepts is one that appears the most obvious and yet, as Lacan was at pains to point out, seems to have been forgotten or ignored by many analysts since Freud: "Whether it wishes to be an agent of healing, training, or sounding the depths, psychoanalysis has but one medium: the patient's speech. The obviousness of this fact is no excuse for ignoring it. Now all speech calls for a response."[5]

---

[2] Jacques Lacan, 'Science and Truth', in *Écrits: The First Complete Edition in English* (New York: W.W. Norton and Company, 2006), 726–45.

[3] Jacques Lacan, *The Seminar of Jacques Lacan Book XIII: The Object of Psychoanalysis*, trans. by Cormac Gallagher (Dublin: http://www.lacaninireland.com, 2011). (Hereafter *Seminar XIII*).

[4] Jacques Lacan, 'The Function and Field of Speech and Language in Psychoanalysis', in *Écrits: The First Complete Edition in English* (New York: WW Norton & Co, 2006), 197–268. (Hereafter 'The Function and Field').

[5] *Ibid.*, 206.

In many ways, the rest of Lacan's very lengthy text can be seen as an unfolding of this basic argument, which appears at the beginning of the first section of the Rome Discourse. And with regards to the importance of speech and language in the constitution of the subject, section two is of particular interest. It is important to point out that Lacan's distinction between 'speech' and 'language' is based on Saussure's distinction between *parole* and *langue*, with the latter representing the 'field of language' (the network of signifiers) and the former representing the way each individual subject utilises this field for their own purposes, which Saussure refers to as the 'psychological' component of language.

Bearing all this is mind, statements such as the following by Lacan provide a very good illustration of the power of language to create a subject:

> Symbols (signifiers) in fact envelop the life of man with a network so total that they join together those who are going to engender him "by bone and flesh" before he comes into the world; so total that they bring to his birth, along with the gifts of the stars, if not with the gifts of the fairies, the shape of his destiny; so total that they provide the words that will make him faithful or renegade, the law of the acts that will follow him right to the very place where he is not yet and beyond his very death; and so total that through them his end finds its meaning in the last judgment, where the Word absolves his being or condemns it...[6]

Taking Lacan's first example, and bearing in mind he was writing in the 1950s, marriage, as precursor to procreation (as it was then likely to be), involves the couple concerned entering into a complex network of signifiers, which include the extended families of the two partners and the marriage ceremony and the legal process of marriage itself. This is the 'discursive world' into which the subject will make their entrance. Furthermore, in many cases the newly born child will have been named before conception, and on arrival into the world is most likely to enter via a complex 'discourse of birth' involving hospitals, midwives, doctors and other medical professionals. In other words, the newly born subject is always already 'caught up' in language.

[6] *Ibid.*, 231.

It is also in this text that Lacan introduces the concept of the Name of the Father, in which, he argues, "…we must recognize the basis of the symbolic function which, since the dawn of historical time, has identified his person with the figure of the law."[7] And he introduces the idea of the *symptom* as "…the signifier of a signified that has been repressed from the subject's consciousness."[8] And perhaps even more significantly, it is in this text that Lacan introduces the idea that "The unconscious is that part of concrete discourse qua transindividual, which is not at the subject's disposal in re-establishing the continuity of his conscious discourse."[9] In other words, the unconscious is not something 'internal' to the individual, but rather a discursive structure. This is the basis of the Lacanian proposition that 'the unconscious is structured as a language'. What this means is that the unconscious is not some 'inner space' that is located somewhere in the human brain, but rather is in the domain of language itself. This is also what allows Lacan to argue, in the Rome Discourse and elsewhere, against the idea of a 'two-body psychology', which is essentially an 'ego-to-ego' (Imaginary) relationship and leads to analysis "…becoming the relation of two bodies between which a fantasmatic communication is established in which the analyst teaches the subject to apprehend himself as an object."[10]

During this period (the early to mid-1950s) Lacan also introduced a number of other key concepts, and one of these was his theory of the object relation in *Seminar IV*.[11] This is important for a number of reasons, not least that in spite of the title of the seminar ('The Object Relation'), Lacan's theory has very little to do with the object relations school of psychoanalysis, which is rooted in the work of Melanie Klein. What Lacan is particularly focused on in the seminar is the question of *lack*, and especially the three different forms of lack of the object. He develops this idea through a close reading of Freud's *Little Hans* case study, and of the three forms of lack he identifies (castration, frustration

[7] *Ibid.*, 230.

[8] *Ibid.*, 232.

[9] *Ibid.*, 214.

[10] Lacan, 'The Function and Field', 251.

[11] Jacques Lacan, *The Object Relation: The Seminar of Jacques Lacan Book IV* (London: Polity Press, 2020).

and privation), *castration* is probably the one that has drawn most attention, and possibly the greatest misunderstanding.

For Lacan, castration is a symbolic operation, that is, it resides in the *Symbolic* register, although its object is in the *Imaginary* register. Lacan states:

> Freud introduced castration in a way that coordinated it fully with the notion of the primordial Law, of the fundamental Law that there is in the incest prohibition and in the structure of Oedipus complex … it was by taking a kind of mortal leap into experience that he (Freud) placed so paradoxical a notion as castration at the heart of the major, decisive and shaping crisis of the Oedipus complex.[12]

Symbolic castration represents the intervention of the law of the signifier into the mother-child 'incestuous' object relation, the 'No' of the Symbolic Father. In the case of Little Hans, the father was a rather ineffectual Father which led to Hans' horse phobia; his fear of the biting (castrating) horse took the place of the absence of the intervention of the Father and thus created the symbolic distance from his mother that is the basis for the resolution of the Oedipal complex. The imaginary object in question here is the Imaginary phallus, the object cause of desire (what Lacan will later formalise as the object *a*) that the child imagines they are for the mother, the object that they believe the mother to be lacking.

At the same time castration represents the expulsion of jouissance, as is indicated in the quote by Lucie Cantin at the beginning of this chapter. Or, to be more precise, it is the replacement of one form of jouissance, which Lacan will later describe as the Other jouissance, by phallic jouissance, which corresponds to Freud's idea of pleasure.[13] In this sense human beings can be said to be 'castrated' by their entry into language, that is, into the Symbolic register. In more Kleinian terms, perhaps, the incestuous and boundaryless relationship of the child with its mother is 'carved up' into clearly defined boundaries structured by symbolic relationships, and in the process a new human subject emerges.

[12] *Ibid.*, 30.

[13] I discuss these forms of jouissance at length in the following chapter.

Bearing all this in mind, and not to mention the twelve seminars Lacan taught prior to *Science and Truth*, why have I chosen this particular text and this particular moment in Lacan's teaching as my 'entry point' into a discussion about the formation of the subject? Primarily, it is because although many of the ideas regarding the relation between the subject of science and the subject of psychoanalysis were present in previous seminars, and especially in *Seminars XI* and *XII*, it is only in *Science and Truth* that, I argue, they come to fruition. It is certainly true that in *Seminar XII, Crucial Problems for Psychoanalysis*[14] that Lacan first posits his idea of the relationship between the emergence of modern science and the Cartesian subject. It is also where he introduces the term 'suture' and where a relatively unknown young French intellectual named Jacques-Alain Miller gives a presentation on that same subject. The concept of suture, as I will argue later on in this chapter, is critical in understanding the nature of the Lacanian subject. However, it is only at the point of *Science and Truth*, in my view, that Lacan makes explicit what he had been leading up to in the two previous seminars: the idea that modern science, that is, a science based on mathematics and mathematical logic, constructs a particular form of human subject, which is also the subject of psychoanalysis. In other words, modern science is what makes psychoanalysis possible; not because psychoanalysis is based on the principles of modern science, but, rather, because of the paradoxical nature of the subject of science itself.

Perhaps another way to look at this is to think of Lacan's teachings between *Seminar I* and *Seminar X* as an exploration and reworking of Freud's key analytic concepts, whereas from *Seminar XI* a more distinctly *Lacanian* theory of the subject starts to be developed which includes situating the emergence of such a subject within a historical context, that of modern science.

It is interesting to note that the particular reading of Lacan that I outlined earlier, that is, the one rooted in the Rome Discourse, the theory of symbolic castration and so on, also seems to equate with what Paul Verhaeghe has described as a 'phallic' reading of Lacan which is designed

---

[14] Jacques Lacan, *The Seminar of Jacques Lacan Book XII Crucial Problems for Psychoanalysis*, trans. Cormac Gallagher (Dublin: http://www.lacaninireland.com, 2011). (Hereafter *Seminar XII*)

to circumvent the question of the Real, jouissance, the drive and object *a*.[15] In this reading, the nearest thing that appears to equate to 'trauma' is (Symbolic) castration, which is an effect of language. But such a 'traumatisation', according to Verhaeghe, is essentially a 'secondary', retroactive phenomenon designed to 'protect' the subject from a more fundamental trauma, which revolves around the drive and the object *a*. If this is the case, then it is difficult to see how this could be described as 'inaugural'. It is only from *Seminar XI* onwards, I argue, as does Verhaeghe in another text,[16] that the emphasis shifts towards this more fundamental trauma.

The Lacanian Subject and the Cartesian Moment

In order to fully appreciate Lacan's reasoning in *Science and Truth* we need to turn to Descartes and the question of knowledge. Descartes' question was, of course, what could he be certain of? Or, to put it another way, having doubted *everything* what was left he could be sure of? And his answer was doubt itself, and although Descartes' famous pronouncement 'I think therefore I am' can be found in Part Four of *A Discourse on Method*[17] the logic behind this is much clearer in his second Meditation:

> But I had the persuasion that there was absolutely nothing in the world, that there was no sky and no earth, neither minds nor bodies; was I not, therefore, at the same time, persuaded that I did not exist? Far from it; I assuredly existed, since I was persuaded. But there I know not what being, who is possessed at once of the highest power and the deepest cunning, who is constantly employing all his ingenuity in deceiving me. Doubtless, then, I exist, since I am deceived; and, let him deceive me as he may, he can never bring it about that I am nothing, so long as I shall be conscious that I am something.[18]

[15] Paul Verhaeghe, 'Subject and Body: Lacan's Struggle with the Real', in *Beyond Gender: From Subject to the Drive*, ed. by Paul Verhaeghe (New York: Other Press, 2001), 65–97.

[16] Paul Verhaeghe, 'Causality in Science and Psychoanalysis', in *Lacan and Science*, ed. by Jason Glynos and Yannis Stavrakakis (London: Routledge, 2002), 119–45.

[17] René Descartes, *A Discourse on Method/ Meditations on the First Philosophy/ Principles of Philosophy* (London: Everyman's Library, 1912).

[18] *Ibid.*, 79–80.

At the beginning of *Science and Truth* Lacan states the following in relation to Descartes:

> ...it might have been noticed that I took my lead last year from a certain moment of the subject that I consider to be an essential correlate of science, a historically defined moment, the strict repeatability in experience which perhaps remains to be determined: the moment Descartes inaugurates that goes by the name *cogito*.[19]

It is perhaps interesting to note that Lacan himself makes reference to the 'inaugural moment' of the *cogito*, but more critical is Lacan's use of the term '*correlate* of science' to describe this 'moment of the subject', rather than simply stating that the Cartesian subject is the 'cause' of modern science. And this touches on a deeper problem: if the Cartesian subject, the *cogito*, is separated from the physical world, that is, the world of the 'hard' sciences (physics, biology, chemistry) then how could such an entity at the same time be a *subject* for such sciences. To gain a better understanding of the problem we need to return to Descartes' mediations and especially *Mediation VI* where he discusses the difference between mind and body. Descartes writes:

> ...although I certainly do possess a body with which I am very closely conjoined; nevertheless, because, on the one hand, I have a clear and distinct idea of myself, in as far as I am only a thinking and unextended thing, and as, on the other hand, I possess a distinct idea of body, in as far as it is only an extended and unthinking thing, it is certain that I [that is, my mind, by which I am when I am] am entirely and truly distinct from my body, and may exist without it.[20]

He goes on to argue that the body is always divisible whereas the mind is not which further reinforces his idea that "...the mind or soul of man is entirely different from the body..."[21] In other words, *cogito* and

[19] Lacan, 'Science and Truth', 727. The reference to 'last year' is to Lacan's previous seminar. The current text is the transcript of Lacan's opening class of his 1965–1966 Seminar on *The Object of Psychoanalysis* (*Seminar XIII*)

[20] Descartes, *Meditations*, 122.

[21] *Ibid*., 128.

corporality are two distinct 'substances' or forms of being. And it is the *corporal* world of physical things that is the subject of the new science, based on mathematics and logic, not the *cogito*.

In chapter 10 of *Lacan, Language and Philosophy*, Russell Grigg explores in some detail the relationship between the Cartesian subject and modern science.[22] He follows Lacan's argument that the birth of modern science is predicated on the birth of the Cartesian subject; however, he makes the further claim, again drawing upon Lacan's arguments, that the Cartesian subject is also the subject of the unconscious, which is essentially the Lacanian subject. In other words, the Cartesian subject equates with the Lacanian subject—or so it would seem. Grigg summarises all this as follows:

> Psychoanalysis he (Lacan) says, would not have been possible without the modern sciences—a general claim that we can break down into at least the two following theses:
>
> The subject on which we operate in psychoanalysis is also the subject of science.
>
> This subject of science is the Cartesian cogito.[23]

However, this should not be interpreted as fulfilling Freud's ambition that psychoanalysis should itself count itself amongst the 'hard' sciences.[24] And neither should it be read as legitimating attempts by some contemporary psychoanalysts (including some within the Lacanian orientation) to somehow 'marry' psychoanalysis with modern neuroscience and cognitive psychology which I referred to earlier. Rather, it is to claim that without modern science, that is, without the emergence of the Cartesian subject, psychoanalysis would not be possible.

In his analysis of this problem Grigg begins by acknowledging that the 'standard' view of Cartesian philosophy is that thought and sensation are

---

[22] Russell Grigg, *Lacan, Language and Philosophy* (New York: State University of New York Press, 2008).

[23] *Ibid.*, 133.

[24] For example, in lecture XXXV of his *New Introductory Lectures*, Freud, in discussing the idea of a *Weltanschauung* for psychoanalysis, concludes by saying: "Psycho-analysis, in my opinion, is incapable of creating a *Weltanschauung* of its own. It does not need to: it is a part of science and can adhere to the scientific *Weltanschauung*. Freud, 'New Introductory Lectures', 181.

not quantifiable and are therefore in the domain of the *cogito*, which in turn frees up mathematics to quantify the physical world through the establishment of natural science. He then goes onto acknowledge that Lacan's claim that the *cogito* is also the subject of science is a radical departure from the 'standard' view. At this point he refers to Lacan's idea in *Science and Truth*, which I have already mentioned, that the Cartesian subject is better understood as the *correlate* of science. According to Grigg, this would mean "…that Lacan's thesis is not a complete revision of the philosophy of science of his mentors, Koyré and Kojève, but rather an attempt to fill out what Lacan thinks it lacks."[25]

But this immediately creates a problem for Grigg's second 'thesis', that is, that the subject of science is the Cartesian cogito. To argue, as Lacan does, that the 'moment' of the Cartesian subject is 'an essential correlate of science', does not, as far as I can see, invalidate the 'standard' view of Cartesian philosophy. To say something is a 'correlate' of something else is simply to posit a *relationship* (which may simply be a statistical one) between one variable and another; it does not, as David Hume recognised nearly three centuries ago, imply *causation*. And it certainly does *not* imply that the Cartesian subject is the subject of science in the sense that the (mathematical and logical) theories and practices of science can be applied to the human subject just as they can to any other 'entity' in the world; the whole point about the Cartesian subject is that it is *excluded* from such theories and practices.

In his discussion of this point Grigg cites Jean-Claude Milner's argument that because the Cartesian subject is devoid of all qualities it is a prime candidate for modern, mathematically based, science. The problem with this argument, according to Grigg, is that it still doesn't address the problem that *res cogitans* (Descartes' 'thinking substance') occupies a completely separate ontological universe to that of *res extensa* (the material world). Milner's problem, argues Grigg, is that "…he assumes that the subject in question must be understood in the following terms: Given that we have science, what must the subject be like that makes this possible?".[26]

---

[25] Grigg, *Lacan, Language and Philosophy*, 137.

[26] *Ibid.*, 145.

However, is this what Lacan actually means by the Cartesian subject being the subject of science? In other words, is Lacan actually arguing that the Cartesian subject, as *res cogitans*, is a subject for scientific study the same way that planets and sub-atomic particles are? I agree with Grigg when he writes that "...what was decisive for the emergence of science was not *just* the constitution of a new object in the form of a mathematized nature but *also* the emergence of the Cartesian cogito as the subject of science."[27] But this is simply a restatement of Lacan's argument that the Cartesian subject is a *necessary condition* for the emergence of modern science, which is very much in line with the 'standard' Cartesian philosophy.

It is important to note that right at the beginning of *Science and Truth* Lacan pays tribute to philosopher of science Alexandre Koyré as being his guide. In fact, Koyré was a key philosophical influence on Lacan's thinking from the 1930s onwards and one of Koyré's main interests was the transition from the medieval worldview to that of modern science. In his book *From the Closed World to the Infinite Universe* Koyré argues that:

> ...the world created by the Cartesian God, that is, the world of Descartes, is by no means the colorful, multiform and qualitatively determined world of the Aristotelian, the world of our daily life and experience—that world is only a subjective world of unstable and inconsistent opinion based upon the untruthful testimony of confused and erroneous sense-perception—but a strictly uniform mathematical world, a world of geometry made real about which our clear and distinct ideas give us a certain and evident knowledge. There is nothing in this world but matter and motion; or, matter being identical with space or extension, there is nothing but extension and motion.[28]

Koyré emphasises a number of times Descartes' contention that God—and the Cartesian cogito—were not part of this world of extension and motion, but, rather, separated from it; the (in)famous 'Cartesian dualism' that philosophers, artists and intellectuals have been struggling with ever

[27] *Ibid.*, 137, italics in original.

[28] Alexandre Koyré, *From the Closed World to the Infinite Universe* (Baltimore: The Johns Hopkins University Press, 1957).

since. There seems little question that the Cartesian universe is very much the basis of the universe of modern science, and especially that of modern physics and cosmology, where everything is quantifiable and articulated in algebraic equations. But at the same time it seems equally obvious that the Cartesian subject has no place *in* this universe, because it lacks 'extension and motion'.

However, it should be noted from Koyré's text that many of the ideas that were essential for the emergence of modern astronomy and physics *pre-dated* Descartes. For example, Koyré pays particular attention to the work of Nicholas of Cusa, the fifteenth century German philosopher and theologian, who was already rejecting the mediaeval conception of the cosmos. He also makes reference to Copernicus, whose seminal work *De revolutionibus orbium coelestium* was published in 1543, to Giordano Bruno, who embraced Copernicanism and paid the ultimate price for doing so by being burnt at the stake in 1600, to Galileo, who was more fortunate, and to Kepler, who Lacan credits with inaugurating the real 'Copernican revolution'.[29] All of these thinkers' ideas pre-date Descartes' *Discourse on Method*, which was published in 1637, and in some cases by over a century. In other words, the conceptual basis for the 'Cartesian' universe was being established *before* Descartes. Therefore, it seems equally as plausible to argue that the 'Cartesian' subject is a *product* of this emerging discourse of science as it is to argue that such a discourse is a product of the emergence of such a subject. Or, to put it another way, 'Cartesian' *science* pre-dates the 'Cartesian' *subject*, insofar as Descartes himself is the embodiment of such a subject.

It is also important to note that in *Science and Truth* Lacan refuses to accept the differentiation between the 'human' and the 'natural' sciences,

---

[29] In *Seminar XX* Lacan states:

> What is crucial, as some people have noticed, is not Copernicus, but more specifically Kepler, due to the fact that in his work it (the Earth in its orbit around the Sun) does not turn in the same way—it turns as an ellipse, and that already throws into question the function of the center. (Jacques Lacan, *The Seminar of Jacques Lacan Book XX 1972–1973: Encore*, ed. by Jacques-Alain Miller (New York: WW Norton & Co, 1999), 43.) (Hereafter *Seminar XX*)

although Lacan prefers the terms 'conjectural' and 'exact' sciences respectively. This matters because it might be thought that even if the 'exact' sciences were not suitable for a 'science of the subject' the 'conjectural' ones might be. This is not to say that Lacan dismisses the importance of the 'conjectural' sciences. On the contrary, he discusses the role of linguistics as a prospective science of the subject and argues that it needs to differentiate "...between the enunciated and enunciation, that is, the impact of the subject who speaks as such (and not of the subject of science)."[30] He goes on to argue that "...one can go very far in the elaboration of the effects of language, since one can construct a poetics that owes no more to references to the mind of the poet than to its incarnation."[31] What Lacan seems to be arguing here is that a theory of the subject is possible within the realms of linguistics which can circumvent the whole question of 'mind' and subjectivity.

This leads Lacan onto a discussion of Lévi-Strauss' structural anthropology (another of his conjectural sciences) which was very influential at the time on Lacan's thinking. Lacan's basic argument is that with the introduction of the concept of the mytheme, Lévi-Strauss was able to create a formalisation of the study of myth. And most critically, in doing so Lévi-Strauss was able to show that:

> The object of mythogeny thus is not linked to any development or stasis of the responsible subject. It is not concerned with this latter subject but rather with the subject of science. And the closer the informer himself is to reducing his presence to that of the subject of science, the more correctly is the collecting [of myth versions] carried out.[32]

Although Lacan does not spell-out what he means by the term 'responsible subject', he appears to be referring to the idea of the 'autonomous individual' beloved of economics (and ego psychology) who is able to exercise 'rational' choices. In fact, such a subject begins to look suspiciously like the Cartesian subject itself. And as Lacan points out, this is *not* the subject of science (or psychoanalysis).

---

[30] Lacan, 'Science and Truth', 731.

[31] *Ibid.*, 731.

[32] *Ibid.*, 732.

It is important to emphasise that Lacan is not looking at psychoanalysis as one discipline amongst many; in other words, as a specific discourse or discursive practice. Rather, he is focusing on the subject of science *as* the subject of psychoanalysis: "This is why it was important to promote firstly, and as a fact to be distinguished from the question of knowing whether psychoanalysis is a science (that is, whether its field is scientific), the fact that its praxis implies no other subject than that of science."[33] This seems to suggest that science *produces* a particular kind of subject which then becomes the focus of psychoanalysis. At this point we need to confront the paradoxical nature of Lacan's argument because he is clearly not talking about *any* subject of science, for example sub-atomic particles, genes, planetary systems, and so on. In fact, from a Cartesian point of view, such entities would be the *objects* of science, not its *subjects*. And as Lacan points out, even psychoanalysis has its own object—the object *a*:

> The object of psychoanalysis (I am laying down my cards now—you may have already guessed my hand, given this talk of the object) is no other than what I have already proposed about the function played in analysis by object *a*. Is knowledge of object *a* thus the science of psychoanalysis?[34]

The answer, according to Lacan, is *no*—the *object a* is not the *subject* of psychoanalysis, its field of study. This is because the object *a* "…must be inserted, as we already know, into the division of the subject by which the psychoanalytic field is quite specifically structured…".[35]

The Sutured Subject

In order to get a better understanding of what Lacan really means by the subject of psychoanalysis it is necessary to examine the concept of *suture*. In the course of a short discussion in *Science and Truth* regarding modern logic Lacan makes the following statement:

[33] *Ibid.*, 733.
[34] *Ibid.*, 733.
[35] *Ibid.*, 733.

> ...Gödel's last theorem (his Incompleteness Theorem) shows that the attempt fails there, meaning that the subject in question remains the correlate of science, but an *antinomic* correlate since science turns out to be defined by the deadlocked endeavour to suture the subject.[36]

The New Oxford English Dictionary defines suture as 'a stitch or row of stitches holding together the edge of a wound or surgical incision' and originates from the Latin *sutura*—'to sew'. And Lacan does use the term in this way a number of times in *Seminar XII*, which is the seminar which immediately proceeds the one for which *Science and Truth* is the first lesson. For example, in his discussion of the construction of the Klein bottle and the torus, which Lacan refers to as 'these little toys', he states that they are constructed through a process of 'vectorialisation': "What does this vectorialisation signify here? That signifies that we construct these figures by a suture, that we stitch what is called here an edge..."[37] Further on Lacan refers to suture as:

> ...an essential buttoning point, which is the one that here opens up a hole, and thanks to which the structure of the Klein bottle is then, and only then, established, namely, that in the sewing which is done at the level of this hole, what is knotted is the surface to itself, in such a way that what we have up to the present taken as outside, is found connected to what we have located up to the present as inside, to what was located as inside, is sutured, knotted to the face that was located up to then as outside.[38]

What's particularly interesting about this passage is that it is at the end of a paragraph which begins by Lacan referring to the emergence of the Cartesian *cogito*, which, according to Lacan, marks the emergence of the psychological subject and the rupturing of the relationship between the subject and cosmos.[39] This rupture then has to be 'stitched up' (sutured),

---

[36] *Ibid.*, 731, my italics.

[37] Lacan, *Seminar XII*, 31.

[38] *Ibid.*, 34.

[39] The complete passage reads as follows:

> The moment of awakening, in so far, as I told you, I highlighted, as I located it historically in the *cogito* of Descartes, is something that is not at all immediately apparent, precisely in the measure that of this *cogito* one makes something that has a psychological value. But if one pinpoints exactly what is in question, if it is what I said, namely the making obvious of the

but the fundamental 'tear' in the fabric of being remains. It is also important to note that Lacan's use of the Klein bottle and the torus are attempts to 'model' the complexities of relating the 'outside', the 'external', to the 'inside', the internal'. I shall return to this question in the concluding chapter.

However, it is Jacques-Alain Miller, in his paper *Suture (elements of the logic of the signifier)*, who gives a more rigorous formulation of the concept of suture and which he defines as:

> ...the relation of the subject to the chain of its discourse; we shall see that it figures there as the element which is lacking, in the form of a stand-in. For, while there lacking, it is not purely and simply absent. Suture, by extension—the general relation of lack to the structure of which it is an element, inasmuch as it implies the position of a taking-the-place-of.[40]

To develop his thesis Miller engages in a detailed analysis of Frege's argument in *Grundlagen der Arithmetik*[41] regarding the genesis of the sequence of whole natural numbers. Miller's is a complex argument which relies on

---

function of the signifier, and is nothing other than the fact that the signifier represents the subject for another signifier, it is starting from this discovery that the supposedly pre-established pact of the signifier with some thing being broken, it is established, it is established in history, and since it is from there that science started, it is established that it is from this rupture, even if immediately, and because simply it is taught only incompletely, and it is taught only incompletely because its final principle is not seen, that it is starting from there that a science can be inscribed, starting from the moment where there is broken this parallelism between the subject and the cosmos which envelopes it, and which makes of the subject, psyche, psychology, microcosm, it is starting from the moment that we introduce here a different suture, and one which I called elsewhere an essential buttoning point, which is the one that here opens up a hole, and thanks to which the structure of the Klein bottle is then, and only then, established, namely, that in the sewing which is done at the level of this hole, what is knotted is the surface to itself, in such a way that what we have up to the present taken as outside, is found connected to what we have located up to the present as inside, to what was located as inside, is sutured, knotted to the face that was located up to then as outside. (Lacan, *Seminar XII*, 34)

[40] Jacques-Alain Miller, 'Suture (Elements of the Logic of the Signifier)', *Screen*, 18.4 (1977), 25–26. Interestingly, a version of this formed a presentation by Miller in Lesson 9 of Seminar XII. However, this section is missing, at least in Gallagher's translation.

[41] Gottlob Frege, *The Foundations of Arithmetic: A Logico-Mathematical Enquiry into the Concept of Number* (New York: Harper & Brothers, 1953).

Frege's idea that the *number* zero is a 'substitute' or 'stand-in' for the *actual* (or in Miller's terminology, *absolute*) zero, that is, nothing. From this proposition Frege claims to be able to generate the whole series of natural numbers. As Miller puts it:

> If of the number zero we construct the concept, it subsumes as its sole object the number zero. The number which assigns it is therefore 1.
>
> Frege's system works by the circulation of an element, at each of the places it fixes: from the number zero to its concept, from this concept to its object and to its number—a circulation which produces the 1.[42]

Frege's construction of the series of natural numbers relies on the differentiation between *concept*, *object* and *number*, and the two operations of (1) the 'subsumption' of the object 'under' the concept and (2) the assignation of a number to the concept.[43] It also relies on the concepts of *identity* and *non-identity*. This allows Frege to define zero as "…the Number which belongs to the concept 'not identical with itself'.[44] This is because *nothing* (as opposed to the *number* zero) 'falls under' the concept 'not identical with itself.' This in turn allows Frege to 'substitute' the number (zero) for the (impossible) object (nothing). Having established zero (as a number) he can then establish the series of natural numbers. As Miller explains:

> Frege's system works by the circulation of an element, at each of the places it fixes: from the number zero to its concept, from this concept to its object and to its number—a circulation which produces the 1.
>
> This system is thus so constituted *with the 0 counting as 1*. The counting of the 0 as 1 (whereas the concept of zero subsumes nothing in the real but a blank) is the general support of the series of numbers.[45]

---

[42] Miller, 'Suture', 30.

[43] For an interesting discussion on this subject see: Erich Reck, 'Frege's Natural Numbers: Motivations and Modifications', in *Gottlob Frege: Critical Assessments of Leading Philosophers, Vol. III*, ed. by Michael Beaney and Erich Reck (Routledge, 2005), 270–301.

[44] Frege, *Foundations of Arithmetic*, 87.

[45] Miller, 'Suture', 30, italics in original.

The generation of the series relies on the *contiguity* of one natural number to another. As Frege puts it:

> There exists a concept F, and an object falling under it *x*, such that the Number which belongs to the concept F is *n* and the Number which belongs to the concept 'falling under F but not identical with *x*' is *m*
> is to mean the same as
> *n* follows in the series of natural numbers directly after *m*.[46]

Or, as Miller explains it, the 'successor' to *n* is $n+1$ which equals ń. This is why, to use Miller's own example, the *number* four is assigned to the *concept* 'member of the series of natural numbers ending with three.'

Miller then goes onto argue:

> In the order of number, there is an addition the 0, and the 0 counts for 1. The displacement of a number, from the function of reserve to that of term, implies the summation of the 0. Whence the successor. That which in the real is pure and simple absence finds itself through the fact of number (through the instance of truth) noted 0 and counted for 1.
>
> Which is why we say the object not-identical with itself invoked—rejected by truth, instituted-annulled by discourse (subsumption as such)—in a word, sutured.[47]

But what has this got to do with the formation (and exclusion) of the subject? At this point, Miller's argument hinges on his introduction of the concepts of metaphor and metonymy, which, although not Lacanian concepts per se, are used extensively in Lacan's theory. Miller argues that the series of natural numbers can be regarded as the 'metonymy of the zero' which relies on the substitution of the *number* zero for the *concept* of zero (nothing) as its starting point. This being the case, Miller then poses the question: "…what is there to stop us from seeing in the restored relation of the zero to the series of numbers the most elementary articulation of the subject's relation to the signifying chain?"[48]

[46] Frege, *Foundations of Arithmetic*, 89.
[47] Miller, *Suture*, 31.
[48] *Ibid.*, 32.

But what is the subject doing here in the first place? As Miller acknowledges earlier on in his paper, the idea of the subject's presence in Frege's logic is something of a paradox because Frege is quite adamant that his theories are not reliant on a human subject. He argues, for example, that: "For a proposition to be true is just not the same thing as for it to be thought."[49] In spite of this Miller is insistent that: "…in the process of the constitution of the series (of natural numbers), in the genesis of progression, *the function of the subject*, misrecognised, is operative."[50] However, Miller is clear that the subject he has in mind is not the *psychological* subject, the subject of modern psychology and psychotherapy (and, it should be noted, the subject of *empiricism*). At the same time, though, Miller is arguing that "…if it is held that the subject is not reducible "…to the psychological, then its *exclusion* from the field of number is assimilable to *repetition*."[51]

Now, it should be clear by now that repetition plays a key role in Frege's generation of the series of natural numbers, because it relies on a series of reiterations starting from zero as a *number*.[52] But in the process of generating this series of numbers, which are also a series of *signifiers*, something, an object, is excluded, which is what Frege defines "not identical with itself."[53] This (impossible) object is the *real* zero (nothing) as opposed to the *number* zero, which, we recall, is the 'stand-in' for the actual, impossible object. And it is this impossible object that Miller names as the *subject*:

> The impossible object, which the discourse of logic summons as the not-identical with itself and then rejects as the pure negative, which it summons and rejects in order to constitute itself as that which it is, which it summons and *rejects wanting to know nothing of it*, we name this object, in so far as it functions as the excess which operates in the series of numbers, the subject.[54]

---

[49] Frege, *Foundations of Arithmetic*, p. 91.

[50] Miller, 'Suture', 27, italics in original.

[51] *Ibid.*, 27, italics in original.

[52] For a useful explanation of this process see: Bird, A. P., 'Frege's Concept Of Natural Numbers', *Medium*, 2021.

[53] Frege, *Foundations of Arithmetic*, 88.

[54] Miller, 'Suture', 32, italics in original.

What Miller is doing here is to demonstrate how it is possible for the subject to both appear and disappear (be excluded) at the same time. But more importantly, he is formulating the *logic of the signifier*, which he defines as "…the relation of lack to the trait (the signifier)."[55] It might be tempting at this point to think that Miller is using Frege's construction of the series of natural numbers out of nothing (so to speak) as an *analogy* to how the human subject both appears in, and is excluded from, the chain of signifiers. However, I am not sure this is what he is getting at. The key thing to remember here is that the subject that both Lacan and Miller are referring to has nothing to do with the subject of psychology or therapy, which is often referred to in terms of the 'self' or the 'ego'. From a Lacanian position, both the 'self' and the 'ego' are products of the *Imaginary*, the *signified*, whereas the subject is a function of the *Symbolic*, the *signifier*. If I understand Miller correctly then what he is arguing is that Frege's logic, that is, the logic that leads to the construction of the series of natural numbers, is *precisely* the logic of the signifier. In the process of suturing, the subject appears both as a *stand-in* (in Fregean logic repeated iterations of zero as *number*) and as *excluded*, the impossible object, which is the subject of the unconscious. This is represented, according to Miller, by $\not{S}A$, which is the subject excluded from the field of the Other.[56]

[55] *Ibid.*, 32. "If we now determine the trait as the signifier, and ascribe to the number the position of the signified, the relation of lack to the trait should be considered the logic of the signifier."

[56] Miller writes:

> What constitutes this relation as the matrix of the chain must be isolated in the implication which makes the determinant of the exclusion of the subject outside the field of the Other its representation in that field in the form of the one of the unique, the one of distinctive unity, which is called 'unary' by Lacan. In his algebra, this exclusion is marked by the bar which strikes the S of the subject in front of the capital A, and which is displaced by the identity of the subject onto the A, according to the fundamental exchange of the logic of the signifier, a displacement whose effect is the emergence of signification signified to the subject. Untouched by the exchange of the bar, this exteriority of the subject to the Other is maintained, which institutes the unconscious. (*Ibid.*, 32–33)

Miller's analysis also throws new light on Lacan's maxim 'the signifier is that which represents the subject for another signifier'.[57] The chain of signifiers is, using Frege's 'model', a series of iterations or repetitions founded on the suturing of the subject. As Miller puts it "…if repetition is produced by the vanishing of the subject and its passage as lack—then only the unconscious can name the progression which constitutes the chain in the order of thought."[58] The reference to 'the order of thought' is significant here because it suggests that a thinking subject is present, in some form, whatever its 'constitution' might be. Miller appears to reiterate this by citing the work of Richard Dedekind, the nineteenth century German mathematician:

> Is it not ultimately to this function of excess that can be referred the power of thematisation, which Dedekind assigns to the subject in order to give set theory its theorem of existence? The possibility of existence of an enumerable infinity can be explained by this, that 'from the moment that one proposition is true, I can always produce a second, that is, that the first is true and so on to infinity.'[59]

However, just to re-emphasise, the subject in question is not the 'self' or 'ego', the *homo psychologicus* as Lacan liked to describe it.[60] The subject in question is excluded from the order of language, the order of signifiers. At the same time there is a 'stand-in' subject, as Miller refers to it, a

---

[57] Lacan makes numerous references to this in his work and in some places compares it to his definition of the sign. For example, in *Seminar XI* he states:

> The whole ambiguity of the sign derives from the fact that it represents something for someone. This someone may be many things, it may be the entire universe, in as much as we have known for some time that information circulates in it, as a negative of entropy. Any node in which signs are concentrated, in so far as they represent something, may be taken for a someone. What must be stressed at the outset is that a signifier is that which represents a subject for another signifier. (Lacan, *Seminar XI*, 207.

[58] Miller, 'Suture', 33.

[59] *Ibid.*, 33.

[60] See, for example, Lacan's *Presentation on Transference*, p. 178 (Lacan, Jacques, 'Presentation on Transference', in *Écrits: The First Complete Edition in English* (New York: W.W. Norton and Company, 2006), 176–85) and *On a Question Prior to Any Possible Treatment of Psychosis*, p. 469 (*Écrits*, 445–88).

subject-as-signifier that makes the whole chain of signification possible. We could think of this as the S_1, the master signifier that 'anchors' the signifying chain.

With regards to the signifier as the subject for another signifier, this has to be read at the level of representation, rather than the excluded subject (the subject of the unconscious). As Miller puts it:

> When Lacan faces the definition of the sign as that which represents something for someone, with that of the signifier as that which represents the subject for another signifier, he is stressing that in so far as the signifying chain is concerned, it is on the level of its *effects* and not of its *cause* that consciousness is to be situated. The insertion of the subject into the chain is representation, necessarily correlative to an exclusion which is a vanishing.[61]

In summary, my argument is that Miller's development of the concept of suture, based on his reading of Frege's theory of natural numbers, is a useful way to conceptualise how the Symbolic order, that is, the network of signifiers, comes into being from 'nothing', so to speak. At the same time, it shows how the subject, somewhat paradoxically, both *appears* in the signifying chain, as a 'stand-in' subject (to use Miller's terminology) and, at the same time, *disappears* under the signifier as the subject of the Real. Furthermore, I argue that Miller's use of Frege's theory of natural numbers should not be taken as an *analogy* for the appearance of the signifying chain and the appearance/disappearance of the subject. Rather, insofar as natural numbers are signifiers themselves, the theory maps out *precisely* how the order of language is generated.

The Cartesian Subject Revisited

At this point it might be helpful to go back to Lacan's original proposition in *Science and Truth* that the 'moment' of the Cartesian subject correlates with the emergence of modern science. The Cartesian subject is

---

[61] Miller, 'Suture', 33, my italics.

what makes modern science, with its focus on quantification, mathematical modelling and so on, possible. But what of human beings themselves? How do they become objects within this Cartesian universe? Clearly, one answer is that they can be studied as physical and biological entities, which is the focus of modern neuroscience and cognitive psychology. And as I touched on earlier there are a number of psychoanalysts who are trying to merge such ideas with those of Freud and other analysts. One of the problems with this approach, however, is that it actually lets the Cartesian subject off the hook, so to speak. In other words, it is quite possible to exhaustively study and conduct experiments upon human brains, the central nervous system, neural networks and so on, whilst still leaving the Cartesian subject intact in its separate universe.

Lacan, on the other hand, is not prepared to let things go so easily. For him, the Cartesian subject is not quite what it seems. And in order to understand why we need to return to Descartes' *cogito, ergo sum* and compare it with Freud's *Wo Es war, soll Ich werden*, which in the Standard Edition is translated as 'where id was, there ego shall be.'[62] In many ways this could almost be regarded as the Freudian version of *cogito, ergo sum*, 'I think, therefore I am', and even in Freud it can read like this. For example, in the Standard Edition reference I just cited, which is at the end of lecture 31 of the *New Introductory Lectures*, Freud states that the aim of psychoanalysis, as a therapeutic endeavour, is:

> ...to strengthen the ego, to make it more independent of the super-ego, to widen its field of perception and enlarge its organization, so that it can appropriate fresh portions of the id. Where id was, there ego shall be. It is a work of culture—not unlike the draining of the Zuider Zee.[63]

This, I would argue, is the psychoanalytic equivalent of the Cartesian cogito: the 'strong ego' looking out into the world, master of all it surveys. This is also the aim of the ego psychology that Lacan spent his whole life battling against; in other words, the purpose of psychoanalysis was seen as the 'strengthening' of the analysand's ego, usually through their identification with the analyst's ego.

[62] See for example Freud's remarks on p.80 in *New Introductory Lectures*.

[63] *Ibid.*, 80.

But what if *Wo Es war, soll Ich werden* can be read a different way? In fact, this is precisely what Lacan does when he interprets it as: "Where it was, there must I come to be a subject".[64] This is probably the nearest Lacan comes to 'defining' the psychoanalytic subject, the *divided* subject, the subject of the *unconscious*. He poses the question: "How could the obscure being, who was [*était*] forever awaiting me, come to be totalized by a line that can only be drawn by dividing this being still more clearly from what I can know of it?"[65] In other words, contrary to Descartes' ascertain that the *cogito* is undivided (only the world of extension can be subject to division) and at the centre of the (epistemological) universe, the Lacanian subject is both divided and decentred.

Furthermore, according to Lacan, *cogito, ergo sum* has to be expressed in *language* for the subject to exist. He argues: "…in the test of writing I am thinking: 'therefore I am,' with quotes around the second clause, it is legible that thought only grounds being by knotting itself in speech where every operation goes right to the essence of language."[66] In other words, it's the *utterance* of 'I think, therefore I am' that brings the subject into being. Although Descartes *wrote* the expression, Descartes himself can only be sure of his existence to the extent he is *speaking* it; otherwise, anyone or thing could have written *cogito, ergo sum*. As Grigg puts it:

> He (Lacan) grants that there is a subject but concludes it is a substanceless subject. Of course, to be able to arrive at this conclusion one has to stop at the evanescent and point-like cogito of the Second Meditation, at the point at which the Cartesian mediator says, " 'I am, I exist' is necessarily true whenever I say it or conceive it in my mind," thus reducing the cogito to its pure utterance.[67]

Clearly, the implication here is that the subject is an effect of language as opposed to Descartes' 'thinking substance.' In fact, Lacan is much clearer about this further on in *Science and Truth* where he states: "Conveyed by a signifier in its relation to another signifier, the subject must be as

[64] Lacan, *Science and Truth*, 734.
[65] *Ibid.*, 734.
[66] *Ibid.*, 734.
[67] Grigg, *Lacan, Language and Philosophy*, 144.

rigorously distinguished from the biological individual as from any psychological evolution subsumable under the subject of understanding."[68] So the subject is neither *res extensa* nor *res cogitans*; rather it emerges within discourse, within the signifying chain (the Symbolic register). And the *process* by which such a subject emerges can be conceptualised by utilising Miller's theory of suture, based around his reading of Frege's theory of natural numbers, that I discussed earlier.

How, though, does this explain Lacan's original proposition that the (divided and decentred) subject of psychoanalysis is the subject of science? In other words, if the 'Cartesian' subject is, in fact, an effect of language, then how did such an effect bring about modern science, because in essence this is Lacan's argument in *Science and Truth*? Perhaps at this juncture we need to change the basic premise of the argument somewhat, having established that the Cartesian subject is not quite as 'Cartesian' as it seems; in other words, there is no rigid demarcation between *res extensa* and *res cogitans* because the *res* in *cogitans* is in fact a *nihil*, so to speak, a no-thing or substance. We also need to remember that Lacan's argument is that there is a *correlation* between the appearance of the Cartesian subject and modern science, not a *causal relationship*. And on this basis it could equally be argued that modern science 'brought about' or made possible the 'Cartesian' subject as much as such a subject 'brought about' modern science. And one of the consequences of the emergence of such a subject is psychoanalysis itself.

Truth, Cause and the Subject of the Real

But what of the truth in *Science and Truth*? So far I have been focusing on the Lacanian subject as the subject of science, but as the title of the text suggests, there is also the question of the subject in relation to truth; or, as we shall see, the subject in relation to the Real. In *Science and Truth* Lacan uses the phrase 'truth as cause' a number of times, especially in his discussion of magic and religion and how they contrast with science. He begins by posing the following question to his audience: "Does or doesn't

[68] Lacan, *Science and Truth*, 743.

what you do imply that the truth of neurotic suffering lies in having the truth as cause."[69] What exactly, though, is Lacan getting at here? Perhaps the first thing to note is that by 'truth' Lacan does not mean *science.* Or perhaps it might be more accurate to say that the kind of truth Lacan is referring to is not the truth of science, and especially modern, Cartesian science. In other words, this is not the truth derived from mathematical theories and experiments.

In the course of his discussion of Freud's *Wo Es war, soll Ich werden* that I referred to earlier, Lacan states that "...nothing gets spoken without leaning on its cause." And, furthermore "...this cause is what is covered (over) by the "*soll Ich*", the "must I", of Freud's formulation, which, in inverting its meaning [*sens*], brings forth the paradox of an imperative that presses me to assume [*assumer*] my own causality."[70] As I understand it, what Lacan means here is that, according to his interpretation of Freud's pronouncement, the *soll Ich* ('must I') is a form of self-causality, as opposed to the subject being 'caused' by some other 'entity'. That Lacan is thinking of Spinoza's concept of self-causation is immediately apparent because he proceeds to argue that:

> The Spinozan self-cause can take on the name of God. It is some-Thing Else [*Autre Chose*]. But let us leave that to the two words I will only play on by stipulating that the Spinozian self-cause is also some-Thing other [*Chose autre*] than the Whole, and that this God, being other in this way, is nevertheless not the God of pantheism.[71]

In Part One of the *Ethics*, Proposition 2, Spinoza states that "Two substances having different attributes have nothing in common with one another."[72] And Proposition 3 states that "If things have nothing in common with one another, one of them cannot be the cause of the other."[73] In other words, by definition everything that is, is self-caused. However,

[69] *Ibid.*, 739. Remember that this paper originally formed the first lesson of Seminar XII; hence Lacan is addressing his question to his audience, many of whom were psychoanalysts.

[70] *Ibid.*, 734.

[71] *Ibid.*, 734–735.

[72] Benedict de Spinoza, *Ethics* (London: Penguin Books, 1996), 2.

[73] *Ibid.*, 3.

this has to be understood within the wider context of Spinoza's argument within the *Ethics*. Essentially, Spinoza is arguing that God is an all-pervading 'substance' that constitutes all of existence. Furthermore, according to Proposition 14 "Except God, no substance can be or be conceived."[74] And, according to Proposition 25 "God is the efficient cause, not only of the existence of things, but also of their essence.",[75]

However, this is not the God of Judeo-Christianity, but rather some form of *pantheistic* entity. As Steven Nadler in his commentary on the *Ethics* points out, Spinoza's 'pantheism', although generally accepted by both his critics and supporters for centuries, can be interpreted in two different ways.[76] Firstly, God and nature are identical; in other words, there is no distinction between God and all there is in the world. This is what Nadler describes as 'reductive pantheism'. On the other hand, there is also the idea that God is distinct from the world and its contents and yet at the same time is 'contained' within it, in the same way that water is contained within a sponge. This is what Nadler calls 'immanentist pantheism' and, he argues, is not a description that can be attributed to Spinoza. On the other hand, he argues, there *may* be a case for describing Spinoza as a 'reductive pantheist', insofar as he equates God with nature.

What is a lot less clear is whether Lacan was thinking in terms of either of these forms of pantheism when he described God as self-cause and at the same time claimed that this was not a pantheistic God. In fact, having just denied that the Spinozian self-cause is the God of pantheism, Lacan then makes reference to the Cartesian *ego* (his term) and the term *ergo* (therefore), which is linked to the concept of cause; as in 'I think, which is caused by/due to my being', although of course this can equally be read as: 'I think therefore I am (caused)', which is the idea, which I referred to earlier, that it is only in speaking that I come into being. According to Lacan:

[74] *Ibid.*, 9.

[75] *Ibid.*, 18.

[76] Steven Nadler, 'Baruch Spinoza', in *The Stanford Encyclopedia of Philosophy*, ed. by Edward N. Zalta, Summer 2022 (Metaphysics Research Lab, Stanford University, 2022). NB: Baruch, Bento and Benedictus are all accepted forms of Spinoza's first name.

> In the *ego* that Descartes accentuates by virtue of the superfluousness of its function in certain of his Latin texts (a subject of exegesis that I leave here to the specialists), one must grasp the point at which it continues to be what it presents itself as: dependent on the god of religion. A curious scrap of *ergo*, the *ego* is bound up with this God. Descartes' approach is, singularly, one of safeguarding the *ego* from the deceitful God, and thereby safeguarding the *ego's* partner—going so far as to endow the latter with the exorbitant privilege of guaranteeing the eternal truths only insofar as he is their creator.[77]

It must be remembered that for Descartes, a devout Catholic, (the Judeo-Christian) God was the ultimate guarantor of existence and certainty. And it is worth pointing out that although Descartes' God appears to be very different from Spinoza's, there are some interesting similarities. Both are the God of Reason, which is the route to salvation (certainty). Both can be 'deduced' from first principles—it should be remembered that Spinoza's *Ethics* is based on a series of axioms and propositions far more elaborate than Descartes'. The critical difference is that whereas Descartes' God occupies the realm of thought (the *cogito*) Spinoza's God is one with Nature.

However, this still doesn't seem to explain Lacan's reference to the Spinozian self-cause as 'some-Thing other than the Whole'. In order to gain a better understanding of what he might be getting at we need to go back to *Seminar XI*. In lesson 2 Lacan states that:

> Cause is to be distinguished from that which is determinate in a chain, in other words the *law*. By way of example, think of what is pictured in the law of action and reaction. There is here, one might say, a single principle. One does not go without the other. The mass of a body that is crushed on the ground is not the cause of that which it receives in return for its vital force … Whenever we speak of cause, on the other hand, there is always something anti-conceptual, something indefinite. The phases of the moon are the cause of tides—we know this from experience, we know that the

[77] Lacan, *Science and Truth*, p. 735.

> word cause is correctly used here. Or again, miasmas are the cause of fever—that doesn't mean anything either, there is a hole, and something that oscillates in the interval. In short, there is cause only in something that doesn't work.[78]

What Lacan is arguing here is that, in both examples (the phases of the moon and miasmas) the word 'cause' does not refer to an actual causal mechanism but a hypothesis or idea (false in both cases). In the first example it is not the phases of the moon that 'cause' the tides but gravitational force; in the second cases it is not 'bad odours' (miasmas) that 'cause' disease but viruses or bacteria. Further on in the seminar Lacan clarifies his distinction between cause and law by making reference to Aristotle's concepts of *tuché* and *automaton*. He begins by arguing that these two words have been incorrectly translated as 'fortune' and 'chance'. He then states that *automaton* equates with the network of signifiers and *tuché* with the encounter with the Real. Before proceeding any further with Lacan's argument it might be helpful to establish how he arrives at this conclusion.

The reference is to Book II of the *Physics*, where Aristotle discusses the four types of cause (αιτία) which are material, form, source, and end. Briefly stated, a material cause refers to what an object is made of, and Aristotle gives the examples of the bronze of a statue or the sliver of a bowl. The form or formal cause refers to the form or pattern of entities and events in the world; Aristotle gives the example of the ratio 2:1 and number in general as the 'cause' of the octave in music. The source refers to what Aristotle describes as the original source of change or rest in an entity or event, for example the person who devises a plan is the 'cause' of its implementation, a father 'causes' the child through its conception. The final cause refers to what we would more likely describe as the aim or objective of a particular action; Aristotle gives the example of health as being the 'cause' of walking (we exercise to be healthy). As William Charlton, in his commentary on Book II of the *Physics*, points out, none

78 Lacan, *Seminar XI*. 22.

of these 'causes' are as straightforward as they might first appear to be,[79] but I do not have the space in this chapter to explore this in more detail.

Aristotle then argues that chance and spontaneity can also be counted as causes. However, at this point, the question of translation becomes crucial. Robin Waterfield, in his translation of the *Physics*, retains the terms 'chance' and 'spontaneity' in the Oxford University Press edition.[80] However, David Bostock, who wrote the Introduction and Explanatory Notes for the same edition, recommends William Charlton's translation, which I referred to above, as staying closest to the Greek phrasing. Charlton argues that in chapter 6 of Book II, Aristotle distinguishes two types of chance: 'luck' (*τύχη*) and 'automaton' (*αὐτόματον*) which he prefers to the more generally used 'spontaneity', although he uses the term 'the automatic' as opposed to 'automaton' for reasons he does not specify.[81]

In chapters 4 and 5 Aristotle spends some time discussing why the concept of chance can be described as a cause in the first place, bearing in mind that: "Some people wonder even whether there are any such things or not. They say that nothing comes to be as an outcome of luck, but that there is a definite cause of everything which we say comes to be as an automatic outcome or as an outcome of luck."[82] On the other hand, he argues that many things occur in life that cannot be attributed to a definitive cause, that is, that are determined, but, rather, they happen by chance. He gives the example of a man going into a market square for some (unspecified) reason but 'by chance' meets another man who owes him money.

Aristotle then goes onto contrast 'luck' with 'the automatic':

> They differ in that the automatic extends more widely. Everything which is the outcome of luck is an automatic outcome, but not everything which is the latter is the outcome of luck. For luck and its outcome belong only to things which can be lucky and in general engage in rational activity.[83]

---

[79] William Charlton, *Aristotle Physics Books I and II* (Oxford: Clarendon Press, 1970). This includes a full translation of the two books along with an extensive commentary and notes.

[80] Aristotle, *Physics* (Oxford: Oxford University Press, 1996).

[81] For the sake of consistency all future references to Books I and II will use Charlton's translation.

[82] *Ibid.*, 31.

[83] *Ibid.*, 36.

What Aristotle is arguing here is that only a rational being can be lucky. This may seem somewhat surprising, bearing in mind that the whole concept of 'luck' (or, to use another term, 'fortune') suggests the *opposite* of rationality and rational explanation. However, what Aristotle is getting at is that luck/fortune can only apply to beings who are able to exercise choice. As Charlton points out, the key point is that Aristotle makes the distinction between those events that are brought about due to the intervention of an external agent ('the automatic') and those that are the result of human choice, even if they were not intended ('luck').

Returning now to Lacan's reading of Aristotle, as I noted earlier he argues that *automaton* and *tuché* have been mistranslated as 'chance' and 'fortune'. Now, it is not clear which translation he is referring to here, but as I pointed out above, the term 'chance', at least according to translators such as Charlton, can mean *both* 'luck' *and* 'automaton'. It's also important to note that *tuché (τύχη) does* translate as 'luck' or 'fortune' according to Liddell and Scott's *Greek-English Lexicon*.[84] Therefore, it is not clear why Lacan objects to this translation.[85]

[84] Henry George Liddell and Robert Scott, *Liddell and Scott's Greek-English Lexicon: Abridged* (Simon Wallenberg Press, 2007). Originally published by Clarendon Press, Oxford, 1909.

[85] In the original (French) version of the seminar Lacan states:

> Ce que j'articulerai la prochaine fois vous montrera comment nous appro prier à ce propos les admirables quatrième et cinquième chapitres de la *Physique* d'Aristote. Celui-ci tourne et manipule deux termes qui sont absolument résistants à sa théorie, la plus élaborée pourtant qui ait jamais été faite de la fonction de la cause—deux termes qu'on traduit improprement par le hasard et la fortune. Il s'agira donc de réviser le rapport qu'Aristote établit entre l'*automaton*—et nous savons, au point où nous en sommes de la mathématique moderne, que c'est le réseau des signifiants—et ce qu'il désigne comme la *tuché*—qui est pour nous la rencontre du réel. (Jacques Lacan, *Le Séminaire de Jacques Lacan: Livre XI Les Quatre Concepts Fondamentaux de La Psychanalyse 1964* (Paris: Éditions du Seuil, 1973), 51)

Compare this with the English version:

> What I will articulate next time will show you how to appropriate to this statement the admirable fourth and fifth chapters of Aristotle's *Physics*. Aristotle turns and manipulates two terms that are absolutely resistant to his theory, which is nevertheless the most elaborate that has ever been made on the function of cause-two terms that are incorrectly translated as *chance* and *fortune*. It is a question, then, of revising the relation that Aristotle establishes between the *automaton*—and we know, at the present stage of modern mathematics, that it is the network of signifiers-and what he designates as the *tuché* which is for us the encounter with the real. (Lacan, *Seminar XI*, 52, italics in original)

However, perhaps what is more important is the *differentiation* between the two terms (*tuché* and *automaton*) in Lacan's argument. In lesson 5 of *Seminar XI* he argues that *automaton* is the "…return, the coming-back, the insistence of the signs, by which we see ourselves governed by the pleasure principle."[86] The *tuché*, by contrast, as an encounter with the Real, is 'beyond' the *automaton*. And, according to Lacan, "The real is that which always lies behind the automaton, and it is quite obvious, throughout Freud's research, that it is this that is the object of his concern."[87] Lacan goes on to argue that *automaton* should not be equated or confused with repetition. This may seem somewhat surprising, bearing in mind his assertion that *automaton* is the 'return, the coming back' of the signifying network, which seems to imply repetition. On contrary, he argues that "What is repeated, in fact, is always something that occurs—the expression tells us quite a lot about its relation to the *tuché—as if by chance*."[88] In other words, the repetition is 'beyond' the signifying network, and, insofar as the signifying network relates to the pleasure principle, 'beyond' the pleasure principle itself. However, is Lacan justified in defining *automaton* and *tuché* in this way? As I noted earlier, in the *Physics* Aristotle argues that that all 'lucky' occurrences fall within the domain of the *automaton*, but not occurrences due to the *automaton* are 'lucky' ones. This in itself is significant because it suggests that, using Lacan's reading, the Real is not 'beyond' the network of signifiers (the Symbolic register) but, rather, *within* it.

But what of the *automaton* itself? In his discussion of the difference between 'luck' and 'the automatic' in Chapter 6, Book II of the *Physics*, Aristotle argues that:

> …in the field of things which in a general way come to be for something, if something comes to be but not for that which supervenes, and has an external cause, we say that it is an automatic outcome; and if such an out-

As can be seen, in the English version *le hasard* is translated as 'chance' whilst *la fortune* is translated as ' 'fortune'. Therefore, the problem (for Lacan) appears to be the initial translations of these terms from the Greek, rather than their French and English equivalents. However, in the text of the Seminar he does not explain the reason for his objection.

86 Lacan, *Seminar XI*, 53–54.

87 *Ibid.*, 54.

88 *Ibid.*, 54 italics in original.

> come is for something capable of choosing and is an object of choice, we call it an outcome of luck.[89]

Charlton, in his commentary on this part of the text, points out that there is a great deal of ambiguity as to whether Aristotle is actually arguing that 'automatic' events are due to nature whereas as 'lucky' ones are due to the actions of rational agents who are capable of exercising choice, that is (for the most part), humans. The two examples that Aristotle uses to illustrate 'the automatic' aren't particularly helpful in this respect. The first is a riderless horse in the midst of battle which 'happens' to find its groom, and the second is a three-legged stool that 'happens' to fall upright and thus provide a seat for someone. With regards to the first example, Charlton argues that although it is possible that the riderless horse would have 'naturally' sought out its rider or groom, it is more likely that the groom or rider sought out the horse. And with regards to the second example, it seems reasonable to assume that the three-legged stool did not 'spontaneously' throw itself up into the air, but, rather, was thrown by someone. In view of this, Charlton suggests that "…a chance doing or undergoing is always one which might have been done due to thought, and it is lucky if done or undergone by a man (sic), and 'automatic' if done or undergone by anything else".[90]

However, none of this seems to help address the question of Lacan's reading of Aristotle, apart, perhaps, from the idea of an 'external' cause. If the *automaton* is associated with the concept of an external cause, this seems to resonate with the idea of the 'external' network of signifiers, which also corresponds to Lacan's concept of the Other (and the unconscious). On the other hand, this still doesn't appear to address the question of the *tuché*; unless, of course, Lacan was picking up on Aristotle's argument regarding the *tuché* as being 'within' the *automaton*, which I referred to earlier. Furthermore, rather than Lacan doing a 'literal' reading of Aristotle regarding the difference between *tuché* and *automaton*, perhaps he was undertaking a more 'structural' reading, where the *differentiation* between the two terms is the critical issue. In this case, what

[89] Charlton, *Aristotle*, 36.
[90] *Ibid.*, 110.

matters is not so much Lacan's understanding of the two concepts per se, but rather his use of them to illustrate the *relationship between* the Symbolic (the *automaton*) and the Real (the *tuché*).

Oliver Harris, in his study of Lacan and antiquity, seems to reach a similar conclusion. He argues that *tuché* and *automaton* both address the question of the *accidental*, with the automaton referring to spontaneous happenings in nature, with tuché as a 'sub-category' of automaton which refer to lucky or unlucky events.[91] In turn, he argues, these can be seen as referring to 'chance for objects' and 'chance for subjects' respectively. Lacan, he argues, uses *automaton* to describe the structural system that produces repetition (which, as we have seen, is *not* what Lacan was arguing) whilst *tuché* refers to the irruption of something else into the realm of *automaton*, which is unassimilable into it. I think his analysis is helpful to the extent that it highlights the *relationship* between *tuché* and *automaton*, which I touched on above, and it does appear to concur, broadly speaking, with Aristotle's argument that *tuché* related to rational beings whereas *automaton* is related to something more 'objective' and 'external'.

Having said that, there are numerous commentaries on Aristotle's concepts of *tuché* and *automaton*, and the broader questions of 'chance' and 'accidents', none of which appear to reach any definitive conclusions on the matter.[92] As James Allen notes:

> "Chance" stands in for the genus designated *αὐτόματον* by Aristotle, which he divides into two species, *τύχη* luck or fortune, which is operative in the realm of practice, and its counterpart in the natural world, the automatic or spontaneous, called, like the genus, *αὐτόματον*. The terminological distinction is stipulative and corresponds neither to Aristotle's own usage nor that of other authors.[93]

---

[91] Oliver Harris, *Lacan's Return to Anitiquity: Between Nature and the Gods* (Abingdon: Routledge, 2017).

[92] Examples include: Licata, Gaetano, 'Aristotle's Doctrine of Causes and the Manipulative Theory of Causality', *Axiomathes*, 29.6 (2019), 653–66; Panayides, Christos, 'Aristotle on Chance and Spontaneous Generation: A Discussion Note', *Filozofia*, 68.2 (2013), 114–23; Massie, Pascal, 'The Irony of Chance: On Aristotle's Physics B, 4–6', *International Philosophical Quarterly*, 43.1 (2003), 15–28; Huismann, Tyler, 'Aristotle on Accidental Causation', *Journal of the American Philosophical Association*, 2.4 (2016), 561–75.

[93] James Allen, 'Aristotle on Chance as an Accidental Cause', in *Aristotle's Physics: A Critical Guide*, ed. by Mariska Leunissen, Cambridge Critical Guides (Cambridge: Cambridge University Press, 2015), 66.

However, Allen also makes the important observation that Aristotle had good reasons to try and address the question of 'chance' in relation to cause:

> ...he (Aristotle) aims to supply an account that will show how chance occurrences can have causes while retaining the distinctive character that sets them apart from their non-chance counterparts. His other main object is to combat on the basis of this account the errors of the natural philosophers who would exclude teleology from physics, replacing explanation in terms of final causes with appeals to chance.[94]

Furthermore, argues Allen, Aristotle is also aiming to undermine those who argue that 'chance' events can be put down to unseen and divine agencies; in other words, they are only 'chance events' from the perspective of human understanding.

But what, then, is Lacan trying to achieve with his references to Aristotle? And more especially, what have such references to do with the foundation of the human subject? Interestingly, Harris points out that Aristotle was not Lacan's only classical reference in *Seminar XI;* he also draws upon Lucretius' reference to the *clinamen* ('swerve', although the modern translation is 'inclination' or 'bias') in *De Rerum Natura.* At the end of lesson 5 Lacan argues:

> If development is entirely animated by accident, by the obstacle of the *tuché*, it is in so far as the *tuché* brings us back to the same point at which pre-Socratic philosophy sought to motivate the world itself.
>
> It requires a *clinamen*, an inclination, at some point.[95]

Now perhaps things start to become clearer: the problem for Lacan is how, in the absence of creationism, is something, in this case the human subject, founded, brought about? Clearly, he could have simply resorted to Darwinism and argued that the human subject is a product of 'natural selection'. However, this would have meant he would have had to revert to some form of biologism or biological determinism, or some

[94] *Ibid.*, 66.

[95] Lacan, *Seminar XI*, 63.

'psychologised' version of this. By referring to Aristotle (and, through Lucretius, the atomism of Democritus, who introduced the concept of the *clinamen*) he is perhaps hoping to avoid any crude form of determinism or reductionism. As I hope is already clear from my discussion above, Aristotle's theory of 'accidental cause', for want of a better term, is anything *but* deterministic or reductionist.

Tuché and the Real

Having established that Lacan had (at least potentially) good reasons for using the concepts of *automaton* and *tuché*, we can now return to his discussion in *Seminar XI* regarding the *tuché* and the Real. In lesson five, following his remarks regarding the *automaton* as the network of signifiers and the Real as that which is 'beyond' the *automaton*, Lacan makes the following statement:

> The function of the *tuché*, of the real as encounter—the encounter in so far as it may be missed, in so far as it is essentially the missed encounter—first presented itself in the history of psycho-analysis in a form that was in itself already enough to arouse our attention, that of the trauma.[96]

Here the relation between *tuché* (as cause), the Real and trauma becomes critical in Lacan's argument. But what exactly is he arguing? That trauma is a missed encounter with the Real? That in a state of trauma the subject somehow 'side steps' the Real? But this is not what Lacan appears to be saying in his seminar. In fact, in lesson five, and especially in his analysis of Freud's 'burning child' dream, it is clear that he is arguing that trauma *is* an encounter with the Real. Furthermore, Jacques-Alain Miller, in his presentation *Psychoanalysis, its place among the sciences*, states that: 'This real of Lacan's, which cannot be said but about which one must speak, is what Freud called 'trauma'. Lacan's real is always traumatic. It is a hole in discourse.'[97]

---

[96] *Ibid.*, 55.

[97] Jacques-Alain Miller, 'Psychoanalysis, Its Place among the Sciences', *Psychoanalytical Notebooks*, 27, 2013, 17.

In order to appreciate what Lacan means by 'a missed encounter' we need to go back a step and explore how Lacan begins in earnest to develop a theory of the Real as a function of language, in the sense of being a 'gap' in the Symbolic order itself, which he does in the first section of *Seminar XI* (lessons two to five). This is also where he develops his theory of the unconscious as an effect of language, rather than being some kind of 'mystical' entity. Even though it could be argued that in this seminar Lacan is at the zenith of his 'structuralist period', at the same time he is already clear that there is a limit to language as a symbolic structure. Perhaps what's particularly interesting in this Seminar is how there appear to be 'two Lacans' rubbing shoulders with one another, so to speak. On the one hand there is the Lacan of the signifier, of the Symbolic; and on the other, the Lacan of jouissance (in the form of the object *a* and the drive), of the Real.

The unconscious occupies a rather contradictory position in all this, because although Lacan speaks of the unconscious as being structured like a language, he also appears to be equating it with the gap in the Symbolic, which is the Real. He talks about the 'pulsation' of the unconscious, of it 'opening' and 'closing'. He goes on to argue that:

> ...the Freudian unconscious is situated at that point, where, between cause and that which it affects, there is always something wrong ... For what the unconscious does is to show us the gap through which neurosis recreates a harmony with a real—a real that may well not be determined.[98]

At this point it becomes difficult, I would argue, to distinguish between the concept of the unconscious and that of the Real. However, one way to differentiate them is to see the unconscious in terms of a structure that *creates* the 'gap' in the Symbolic that Lacan will name as the Real:

> Impediment, failure, split. In a spoken or written sentence something stumbles. Freud is attracted by these phenomena, and it is there that he seeks the unconscious. There, something other demands to be realized—which appears as intentional, of course, but of a strange temporality. What

[98] Lacan, *Seminar XI*, 22.

> occurs, what is *produced*, in this gap, is presented as *the discovery*. It is in this way that the Freudian exploration first encounters what occurs in the unconscious.[99]

Here Lacan refers to what *occurs in* the unconscious, what is *produced* in the gap. The 'hole' in the Symbolic is structural and subject to the laws of the signifying chain, but what is 'in' the hole is not. Lacan also refers to the gap of the unconscious as being pre-ontological, which means that it belongs to the order of the *unrealised* as opposed to *non-being*. With regards to the *discovery*, as Lacan points out, this is essentially as *re*discovery, which 'is always ready to steal away again, thus establishing the dimension of loss.'[100] Just as soon as the unconscious opens up it closes again, and what is lost is the object *a*, which in *Seminar X* Lacan had already established as the object cause of desire,[101] and which later on he will refer to as surplus jouissance, a piece of the Real.

Further on in *Seminar XI* Lacan argues that transference to the subject-supposed-to-know is the response of the subject's encounter with trauma:

> One may go so far as to believe that the opacity of the trauma—as it was then maintained in its initial function by Freud's thought, that is to say, in my terms, its resistance to signification—is then specifically held responsible for the limits of remembering. And, after all, it is hardly surprising, given my own theorization, that I should see this as a highly significant moment in the transfer of powers from the subject to the Other, what I call the capital Other (*le grand Autre*), the locus of speech and, potentially, the locus of truth.[102]

Lacan argues that the Other, the subject-supposed-to-know, is already present in the opening of the unconscious, 'however fleeting it may be'. Essentially, the transference is 'the means by which the communication

[99] *Ibid.*, 25, italics in original.

[100] *Ibid.*, 25.

[101] Jacques Lacan, *The Seminar of Jacques Lacan: Book X: Anxiety 1962–1963* (Cambridge: Polity Press, 2014). (Hereafter *Seminar X*)

[102] Lacan, *Seminar XI*, 129.

of the unconscious is interrupted'.[103] Pierre-Gilles Guéguen, in his paper *Paradoxes of the Births of Transference*, reinforces Lacan's argument that transference occurs at the very moment of the encounter of the subject with the Real, with the trauma. As Guéguen explains:

> Lacan's expression "closing of the unconscious" in this context designates the fact that in transference the subject gives meaning back to what was disturbed. The subject forgets that he is but the effect of the signifying chain, that he is only its remainder, re-woven with the Symbolic and the Imaginary that for an instant becomes undone. *The clinic of trauma gives us the most striking example of this.*[104]

Guéguen cites the example of Freud's text on the Acropolis where he experienced a momentary sense of depersonalisation. He 'resolves' this loss of meaning by 'spinning the story of the rivalry with his father and his guilt at having socially "surpassed" him.'[105] In other words, the intervention of the Other is enough to bring Freud back to 'reality', that is, the Symbolic-Imaginary matrix. In this sense the encounter with the Real is not so much *missed* as *avoided*; the trauma of the Real is too much for the subject to bear so there is a 'transfer' to the Other.

And yet, somewhat paradoxically, Lacan also argues in *Seminar XI* that "...the transference is the enactment of the unconscious."[106] Furthermore, such an unconscious is consubstantial with sexuality. In another paper Guéguen point outs that in *Seminar XI* "...Lacan announces that while transference closes up the unconscious, repetition—somewhat surprisingly—allows for its opening."[107] This makes it clear that, for Lacan at least, transference should not be seen as a 'repetition' in the analytic setting of the subject's earlier relationships, for example with his or her parents. Instead, as Guéguen explains, Lacan "...focuses the attention on the

---

[103] *Ibid.*, 130.

[104] Pierre-Gilles Guéguen, "Paradoxes of the Births of Transference," *Psychoanalytical Notebooks*, no. 17 (March 2008): 41–45.

[105] *Ibid.*, 43.

[106] Lacan, *Seminar XI*, 146.

[107] Pierre-Gilles Gueguen, "Transference: A Paradoxical Concept," *LC Express* 2, no. 12 (December 2014), 4.

type of repetition that opens up to the unconscious as trauma because it unceasingly indicates how the subject defends himself from the real, how he avoids it."[108] And the subject avoids the Real through…the transference. So what we have here is strange type of dynamic (or dialectic) involving the perpetual 'missing' of the subject's encounter with the Real: at the moment of the subject's encounter with the Real, there is a move (a 'transfer') to the Symbolic.

At the same time, this is *always* a missed encounter for quite 'structural' reasons. As Lacan notes in lesson five of *Seminar XI,* just after his remarks about *tuché* and the missed encounter with the Real: "Is it not remarkable that, at the origin of the analytic experience, the real should have presented itself in the form of that which is *unassimilable* in it—in the form of the trauma, determining all that follows, and imposing on it an apparently accidental origin?"[109] In other words, the Real, in the form of trauma, cannot be symbolised, cannot be assimilated into the Symbolic order. So structurally there a 'gap', a void, in the fabric of 'reality', that is, in the network of signifiers. Essentially, the subject 'encounters' an *absence.* Furthermore, and referring back to Miller's arguments regarding suture, it could perhaps equally be argued that the *subject itself* is this absence; and insofar as this absence is the Real, which can in turn be equated with trauma, then it could be argued that the subject, which is perpetually 'vanishing' within the network of signifiers, is *trauma itself.*

Conclusion: The Emergence of the Lacanian Subject

Contrary to what can sometimes appear to be an 'ahistorical' reading of Lacan, that is, the impression that the subject simply 'appears' in an ever-present linguistic framework, if we follow Lacan's argument in *Science and Truth* then it is clear that the Lacanian subject emerges at a very specific moment in history; or, to be more precise, it emerges within a very specific *discourse.* This is the discourse of *science* and, more

[108] *Ibid.*, 5.

[109] Lacan, *Seminar XI*, 55, italics in original.

specifically, the discourse of *mathematical* science, which can also be referred to as *modern* science. Although often associated with Descartes, as I have argued in this chapter many of the ideas that underpin modern science pre-date him. It is also perhaps worth noting, as does Koyré, that the Cartesian world view has since been superseded by others, most notably Newton's, and, more recently, Einstein's and that of the quantum physicists. However, these frameworks are still very much reliant on mathematics and modern logic, so perhaps in a looser sense they can still be described as 'Cartesian'.

Returning to Lacan's idea in *Science and Truth* of truth as cause, I would like to propose that the 'cause' in question is the Real, which can also be seen as *trauma*, and, in many ways, the subject itself. This is the 'truth' of the subject; a subject sutured by the language of science, and which emerges as the subject of psychoanalysis. Although such a subject could broadly be described as 'Cartesian', as Lacan is at pains to argue (particularly in *Science and Truth*, but also in many other parts of his work), this 'Cartesian' subject is not quite what it seems. In fact, it is a total paradox, because it both exists within the chain of signifiers and, at the same time, is completely absent. The 'Cartesian' subject is a *sutured* subject—a 'stand-in', a *fabrication*, which hides the absence of the Real subject. And yet, even more paradoxically, the truth of the subject is *precisely* this absent, Real, subject, which even though it may not ek-sist,[110] perpetually *in-sists*.

But this is by no means the end of the story; in fact, it is only the beginning. The discourse (*automaton*) of science is not a 'fixed' entity, but rather an ongoing, 'dynamic' force, as are its traumatising effects. In other words, trauma is not a 'one-off' event that 'inaugurates' the subject, but rather a continuous process, which is linked very closely to the Freudian concept of the *drive* and to Lacan's concept of *jouissance*. And it is to these ideas that we must now turn.

[110] In the Heideggerian sense of to 'stand-out from oneself'. For a useful discussion of the term 'ek-sistence' see Kevin Aho's entry in *The Cambridge Heidegger Lexcicon* (Cambridge University Press, 2021), 268–270.

5

From Trauma to Drive-Jouissance

The Drive: Introductory Remarks

In the previous chapter I explored the idea that the subject is constituted or 'inaugurated' by the entry of the human being into language; and more specifically, by their entry into the language of science. This is a paradoxical, divided and 'sutured' subject that is both a 'stand-in' subject of language and a subject of the Real. As a subject of the Real the subject *is* trauma. However, I also pointed out in my concluding remarks that this is not a 'once and for all' trauma; rather, it is a 'dynamic' trauma in the sense that the subject is being continually 'subjected' to the operation of the drive. In this chapter I want to spend some time exploring this concept and especially how it relates to jouissance and trauma.

I begin by examining Freud's theory of the drive, which is given the most comprehensive articulation in *Instincts and their Vicissitudes*, and then discuss Lacan's 'deconstruction' of Freud's theory in *Seminar XI*. I then go on to explore Lacan's theory of jouissance within the framework of Miller's 'six paradigms' followed by an exploration of Miller's concept of an embodied jouissance. I conclude by discussing how these ideas

© The Author(s), under exclusive license to Springer Nature Switzerland AG 2025

L. Chapman, *Traumatic Neurosis Revisited*, The Palgrave Lacan Series,
https://doi.org/10.1007/978-3-031-89158-8_5

can be used to construct a theory of trauma based on the jouissance of the drive, and, more specifically, surplus jouissance.

Before proceeding with my main argument I would like to briefly address a rather fundamental issue of translation: the use of the word 'instinct' instead of 'drive' in Strachey's *Standard Edition*. As a number of commentators have pointed out, not least Lacan himself,[1] this decision to translate the German *Trieb* as 'instinct' is somewhat unfortunate because of its biological implications, even though, as we shall see shortly, Freud was very clear that *Trieb* meant something else entirely. Strachey's rationale for his decision can be found in his General Introduction to *The Standard Edition*.[2] The crux of his argument is that the term 'drive', in the way it is used in Freud's work, is not one to be found in the large Oxford English Dictionary or in any English psychology textbooks of the time of publication of the General Introduction (1966). Furthermore, Strachey notes that Freud uses the term *Trieb* in at least three different ways, and his argument is that:

> It is not the business of a translator to attempt to classify and distinguish between Freud's different uses of the word. This job can safely be left to the reader, provided only that the same English word is invariably used for the German original ... The only rational thing to do in such a case seems to me to be to choose an ***obviously vague and indeterminate word*** and stick to it.[3]

At the same time, though, Strachey notes that Freud on occasion uses the word *Instinkt* in relation to animal biology, which implies that he viewed *Trieb* as something non-biological. With regards to the problems of translation, Strachey's argument that because the term *Trieb* has multiple meanings and, furthermore, its translation as 'drive' might be unfamiliar to non-German speakers, and therefore it is better stick to a 'vague and indeterminate word', seems very weak and somewhat peculiar. Perhaps it might be better, in fact, to leave the term in its original language.

[1] See for example his comments regarding Strachey's translation of *Trieb* as 'instinct' in *Seminar XI*, 49.

[2] James Strachey, "Some Technical Terms," in *The Standard Edition*, vol. I (London: Hogarth Press, 1966), xxiii–xxvi.

[3] *Ibid.*, xxv, my italics.

And at this point it is also worth noting Rolf Flor's arguments regarding the issue of translation and especially the idea that much of the time the word Trieb appears in Freud's writing as part of much larger composite words, for example *Sexualtreibe*, *Destruktiontriebe*, *Erhaltungtriebe*, and so on. According to Flor this is because Freud:

> ...*is struggling to explain exactly what he is saying.* What determines the drive notion in general that he would like to clarify? What kinds of drives can there be? He is literally tying *Trieb* to so many other concepts in order to help the reader and *perhaps even to clarify the notion for himself!* [4]

In other words, it is not simply a problem of translation; rather, there appears to be a more fundamental conceptual problem here, that is, the precise nature of the drive itself. On the other hand, it could be argued that it is precisely this impreciseness that gives the concept its strength because it allows a degree of flexibility in its use; something that is particularly useful when it comes to thinking about the 'extimacy' of the drive.

The other important point to note at this stage is that I will be using the term 'drive' (singular) whenever possible rather than 'drives' (plural).[5] This is essentially a Lacanian convention and one of the reasons it is used is because Lacan argues in a number of texts and seminar lessons that, ultimately, every drive is a death drive.[6] This is to do with the idea of the drive as *repetition*, continually circling around the object *a*, and is something I discuss later on in this chapter.

---

[4] Rolf Flor, "On the Very German-Ness of Freud's Trieb," in *Critical Essays on the Drive: Lacanian Theory and Practice*, ed. Dan Collins and Eve Watson, The Lines of the Symbolic in Psychoanalysis Series (Abingdon, Oxon: Routledge, 2024), 50, italics in original.

[5] The only exceptions are when the term 'drives' is used in quoted text or when it is clear that the author I am referring to is using the plural form, for example when referring to the partial *drives*.

[6] For example, in 'Position of the Unconscious', during his discussion of the concept of the lamella, Lacan states:

> Speaking subjects have the privilege of revealing the deadly meaning of this organ, and thereby its relation to sexuality. This is because the signifier as such, whose first purpose is to bar the subject, has brought into him the meaning of death. (The letter kills, but we learn this from the letter itself.) This is why every drive is virtually a death drive. Jacques Lacan, 'Position of the Unconscious', in *Écrits: The First Complete Edition in English* (New York: W.W. Norton and Company, 2006), 719.

Freud and 'Instincts and Their Vicissitudes'

Although, as Laplanche and Pontalis point out, the term *Trieb* (drive) first appears in Freud's *Three Essays on the Theory of Sexuality* along with his distinction between the source, object and aim of the drive,[7] it is in his 1915 paper *Instincts and their Vicissitudes* where Freud fully formulates his theory. Therefore, any discussion on drive theory needs to begin with this text, especially as Lacan makes extensive reference to it in his 're-reading' of Freud's drive theory in *Seminar XI*.

Freud begins by pointing out the difference between a drive and a stimulus:

> In the first place, an instinctual stimulus (drive) does not arise from the external world but from within the organism itself ... all that is essential in a stimulus is covered if we assume that it operates with a single impact, so that it can be disposed of by a single expedient action ... An instinct, on the other hand, never operates as a force giving a *momentary* impact but always as a *constant* one.[8]

As Freud notes, one of the problems with such a constant, internal force is that the organism cannot escape from it, unlike the case with an external stimulus/threat. Therefore, the organism's nervous system (Freud's terminology which Lacan names the *Real Ich*) has to develop ways to 'regulate' this constant excitation that originates from 'within'. In a footnote Strachey notes that this idea of 'regulation' is the basis of the 'principle of constancy, which appears in some of Freud's earliest writings.[9] And as I noted in Chap. 3, this is also linked to Freud's concept of the pleasure principle.

Freud goes onto argue that another way of looking at the drive is as a *frontier* concept:

[7] Laplanche and Pontalis *The Language of Psychoanalysis*, 215.

[8] Freud, 'Instincts and Their Vicissitudes', 118, italics in original.

[9] *Ibid.*, 119.

> …an 'instinct' appears to us as a concept on the frontier between the mental and the somatic, as the psychical representative of the stimuli originating from within the organism and reaching the mind, as a measure of the demand made upon the mind for work in consequence of its connection with the body.[10]

In other words, a *drive* is not the same as a biological *instinct*, even though Freud claims to be borrowing the concept from biology and applying it to the psyche. However, the idea of the drive as a 'psychical representative' is not itself without problems. As Laplanche and Pontalis note, Freud seems to be using the term to mean a *somatic delegation* within the psyche, but in fact he uses this concept of 'delegation' in two different ways.[11] Firstly, in the manner described in the above quote, that is, "…as the psychical representative of the stimuli originating from within the organism and reaching the mind." Secondly, as in its use in Freud's *Repression* paper, where he refers to the repression of an 'instinctual representative' which, according to Freud, is "…an idea or group of ideas which is cathected with a definitive quota of psychical energy (libido or interest) coming from an instinct."[12] However, as Freud immediately points out, this means the drive is part idea (*Vorstellung*)[13] and part 'quota of affect'. Repression, he argues, means "…we shall have to follow up separately what … becomes of the *idea*, and what becomes of the instinctual energy linked to it."[14] According to Laplanche and Pontalis, this second formulation implies that the drive is "…part of the process of somatic excitation.",[15] whereas this is lacking in the first formulation. However, they argue that these two formulations are not contradictory: "Since this relation is constant in Freud's propositions we may reasonably assume that the difference between them is merely semantic."[16]

---

[10] *Ibid.*, 121–122.

[11] Laplanche and Pontalis, *The Language of Psychoanalysis*, 364–365.

[12] Sigmund Freud, 'Repression', in *The Standard Edition of the Complete Psychological Works of Sigmund Freud* (London: Hogarth Press, 1915), V, 152. It is not clear whether in this context Freud is referring to *Trieb* or *Instinkt*.

[13] Although Laplanche and Pontalis opt for 'ideational representative' (*Vorstellungsrepräsentanz*).

[14] Freud, 'Repression', 152, italics in original.

[15] Laplanche and Pontalis, *The Language of Psychoanalysis*, 364.

[16] *Ibid.*, 365.

Having defined the drive as a frontier concept Freud then outlines the four key 'components' of the drive: its pressure (*Zang*), its aim (*Ziel*), its object (*Objekt*), and its source (*Quelle*). This decomposition of the drive allows Freud (and Lacan) to argue that the paths to satisfaction of the drive (its aim) can vary considerably as can its object. As Freud points out, the object of the drive:

> …is what is most variable about an instinct and is not originally connected with it, but becomes assigned to it only in consequence of being peculiarly fitted to make satisfaction possible. The object is not necessarily something extraneous: it may equally well be a part of the subject's own body.[17]

It is interesting to note, perhaps, that Freud leaves the question of the drive's *source* until last, even though this might be thought of as the most important aspect of all. He argues that the source of the drive refers to, "…the somatic process which occurs in an organ or part of the body and whose stimulus is represented in mental life by an instinct (drive)".[18] Earlier on in the paper Freud makes reference to *instinctual stimuli*, which originate from within the organism, and which cannot be mastered by a simple flight or fight mechanism. In fact, argues Freud, such stimuli, because they maintain an "…incessant and unavoidable afflux of stimulation", cannot even be regulated by the nervous system in the way other, external, stimuli are dealt with through the principle of constancy. Although Freud is not explicit at this point about the nature of such instinctual stimuli, they would appear to be biological.

Freud proposes that although there may appear to be many types of drives, they can ultimately be reduced to two 'primal' ones: the *ego* or *self-preservative* and the *sexual* drives, although, in *Beyond the Pleasure Principle* this idea undergoes a radical revision with the introduction of the death drive.

Coming now to the vicissitudes (changes) mentioned in the title of his paper, Freud argues that there are four main ones:

---

[17] Freud, 'Instincts and their Vicissitudes', 122.

[18] *Ibid.*, 123.

1. Reversal into its opposite.
2. Turning round upon the subject's own self.
3. Repression.
4. Sublimation.

In his paper Freud focuses on the first two vicissitudes, and with regards to the reversal of the drive into its opposite, he argues that this can be further broken down into a change from activity to passivity, and a reversal of content. He uses the examples of two pairs of opposites, sadism-masochism and scopophilia-exhibitionism to illustrate the reversal from activity to passivity, and the transformation of love into hate to illustrate the reversal of content.

Freud spends some time discussing the vicissitudes of love in the final section of his paper. He argues:

> The case of love and hate acquires a special interest from the circumstance that it refuses to be fitted into our scheme of the instincts. It is impossible to doubt that there is the most intimate relation between these two opposite feelings and sexual life, but we are naturally unwilling to think of love as being some kind of special component instinct of sexuality in the same way as the others we have been discussing. We should prefer to regard loving as the expression of the *whole* sexual current of feeling; but this idea does not clear up our difficulties, and we cannot see what meaning to attach to an opposite content of this current.[19]

The gist of Freud's argument here is that unlike the 'opposites' sadism-masochism and voyeurism-exhibitionism, the opposition love-hate is more complicated. As Freud puts it, there is the opposition loving-hating, but also loving-being loved, and, furthermore, loving/hating-indifference (which would not apply to the other two examples). Freud argues that the second opposition (loving-being loved) corresponds to the transformation from activity to passivity, which also applies to sadism-masochism and scopophilia-exhibitionism. This is rooted in the idea of loving oneself (narcissism) but undergoes a transformation into loving an external

[19] *Ibid.*, 133, italics in original

object (person), which is an active position or being loved by an external object (a passive position).

At this point Freud introduces what he describes as the 'three polarities' which govern mental life: subject (ego)—object (external world); pleasure-unpleasure; active-passive. Freud makes an interesting observation regarding the first 'polarity', which is that whereas the individual organism can escape from *external* stimuli by movement it cannot do so with regards to *internal* stimuli.[20] In other words, it is the stimuli (excitations) of the drive that becomes particularly problematic for the subject.

He goes onto argue that the polarities ego-object and pleasure-unpleasure coincide at the earliest point in the development of mental life, which is when the ego is cathected (energised) with the drives and is able to satisfy them itself; this is the state of *narcissism* and the ego's method of drive satisfaction is *auto-erotic*. Freud points out that "At this time the external world is not cathected with interest ... and is indifferent for purposes of satisfaction."[21] This means that, from the ego's point of view, only the 'internal' world (which coincides with the ego itself) is deemed pleasurable whereas the 'outside' world is either viewed with indifference or as unpleasurable (to the extent it is a source of unwelcome stimulation/excitation).

As Freud points out, the ego as auto-erotic does not require an external world, but in order to survive it needs to 'acquire' objects from that world. Because of this"... it (the ego) cannot avoid feeling internal instinctual stimuli for a time as unpleasurable."[22] At this point, "under the dominance of the pleasure principle", objects that are deemed pleasurable by the ego are *introjected* (taken into itself) whereas those that are deemed unpleasurable are expelled through the mechanism of *projection*. In the process the 'reality-ego' becomes a 'pleasure-ego', and the 'external' world becomes hostile and is equated with unpleasure.

Freud goes onto argue that *loving* an object more and more refers to any object that satisfies the ego, which is not the same as 'needing' it (which equates with self-preservation). In particular, such love refers to

[20] *Ibid.*, 134.
[21] *Ibid.*, 134–135.
[22] *Ibid.*, 135,

objects that bring *sexual* satisfaction. *Hate*, on the other hand, is focused on those objects which bring 'unpleasure':

> The ego hates, abhors and pursues with intent to destroy all objects which are a source of unpleasurable feeling for it, without taking into account whether they mean a frustration of sexual satisfaction or of the satisfaction of self-preservative needs. Indeed, it may be asserted that the true prototypes of the relation of hate are derived not from sexual life, but from the ego's struggle to preserve and maintain itself.[23]

This differentiation between 'internal' and 'external' and their relation to objects of love and hate is important because it suggests that the whole concept of 'internal-subjective' versus 'external-objective' is by no means a 'given' in the life of the subject. As I explain in the Conclusion, this is something Lacan attempts to address with his concept of 'extimacy' and various topological figures such as the möbius strip and the torus that are used to illustrate the continuity rather than the discontinuity between 'internal' and 'external'.

Lacan's 'Deconstruction' of the Drive[24]

Although Freud was to go onto radically modify his theory of the drive in *Beyond the Pleasure Principle* his paper *Instincts and their Vicissitudes* is still a key reference point, especially for Lacan in *Seminar XI*. It is also in this seminar that Lacan further develops his concept of the object *a* which will become pivotal in his later work when he explores the relationship between the drive and jouissance. Therefore, I will devote the next part of this chapter to a fairly detailed analysis of Lacan's arguments regarding the drive. The three lessons in the Seminar that are especially pertinent are 'The Deconstruction of the Drive' (lesson 13), 'The Partial Drive and

[23] *Ibid.*, 138.

[24] It is important to note that although Lacan uses the term 'deconstruction' when referring to the drive, he is not using it in the philosophical (e.g. Derridean) sense of the term. Rather, he is developing Freud's idea that the drive has a number of different 'components', i.e. source, object, aim and thrust. I have retained the word 'deconstruction' only because of Lacan's use of the term.

its Circuit' (lesson 14), and 'From Love to the Libido' (lesson 15). Where appropriate I will also draw upon Philip Dravers' commentary which gives a Millerian perspective on this part of the Seminar.[25]

Lacan begins his discussion by reminding his audience that the drive has to be conceived of as a constant force (*konstante Kraft*) as opposed to a shock force or some form of kinetic energy. This leads Lacan to conclude that the drive cannot be seen in terms of a biological function, which would always have a rhythm. This is also a reminder that the drive should not be confused with the instinct. Dravers, drawing upon Miller's arguments, notes that the instinct can be thought of as a 'program' operating in the Real, whilst the drive is a constant (non-biological) force:

> The drive … is not something that arises at the level of a biological need; it is not of the order of hunger or thirst, appearing on the basis of the natural rhythms of the body. It has no 'natural' object that could appease its tension, but emerges as a constant force, a *konstante Kraft* to use Freud's term, that expresses itself as a continual demand for satisfaction.[26]

The drive can be seen as a rupture in the natural order and as the basis for history and civilisation. It installs itself in the living being through the effects of language on the body. As I commented upon in the latter part of Chap. 3, this link with history is something Lacan touches upon in his commentary on the death drive in *Seminar VII*, which I will return to later in this chapter.

With regards to the aim of the drive, Lacan questions whether this equates with satisfaction, focusing particularly on one of Freud's four vicissitudes—sublimation.[27] The point about sublimation, he argues, is that "…Freud tells us repeatedly that sublimation is also satisfaction of the drive, whereas it is *zielgehemmt*, inhibited as to its aim – it does not attain it."[28] However, Lacan then suggests that in fact satisfaction *does*

---

[25] Philip Dravers, "The Drive as a Fundamental Concept of Psychoanalysis," *Psychoanalytical Notebooks*, no. 23 (September 2011): 117–49.

[26] *Ibid.*, 123.

[27] According to Freud there are four vicissitudes—reversal into its opposite; turning around upon the subject's own self; repression; sublimation (Freud, 'Instincts and their Vicissitudes', 126).

[28] Lacan, *Seminar XI*, 165.

equate with the aim; he cites the examples of patients who gain satisfaction from their symptoms, even when these appear to produce displeasure. "One cannot say, then, that the aim is not attained where satisfaction is concerned. It is."[29] But this satisfaction is paradoxical: "The path of the subject—to use the term in relation to which, alone, satisfaction may be situated—the path of the subject passes between the two walls of the impossible."[30]

And he defines this impossible as the Real, arguing that it is an obstacle to the pleasure principle, although he then goes onto argue that the impossible is present in the field of the pleasure principle itself, in the sense that the drive can never reach satisfaction:

> By snatching at its object, the drive learns in a sense that this is precisely not the way it will be satisfied. For if one distinguishes, at the outset of the dialectic of the drive, *Not* from *Bedürfnis*, need from the pressure of the drive—it is precisely because no object of any *Not*, need, can satisfy the drive.[31]

He then introduces the object *a*,[32] the object cause of desire, into the argument, and using the example of the mother's breast as the object *a*, states that its place in the satisfaction of the drive can be thought of as *la pulsion en fait le tour*. In a footnote to the text Alan Sheridan, the translator, explains that what Lacan is getting at here is that the drive both moves around the object and 'tricks' it. By 'trick' what Lacan appears to mean is that the drive 'tricks' the subject into thinking the *actual* object, in this case the mother's breast, is *the* (lost) object, the object *a*. Dravers' perspective on this is that the 'trick' of the drive refers to the 'capturing' of a piece of the Real in the form of the object *a*. It is only through the

[29] *Ibid.*, 166.

[30] *Ibid.*, 167.

[31] *Ibid.*, 167.

[32] In different Lacanian texts there are different ways of writing the English translation of *objet petit a*. Some authors choose object a (without any italicisation), others *object a* (with italics) and others object *a*, which is my preferred rendering of the term.

drive that psychoanalysis can have an effect on the Real in the field of transference.[33]

Lacan then moves on to discuss the source of the drive. In *Instincts and their Vicissitudes* Freud states the following:

> By the source [*Quelle*] of an instinct is meant the somatic process which occurs in an organ or part of the body and whose stimulus is presented in mental life by an instinct...Although instincts are wholly determined by their origin in a somatic source, in mental life we know them only by their aims. An exact knowledge of the source of an instinct is not invariably necessary for the purpose of psychological investigation; sometimes its source may be inferred from its aim.[34]

In his seminar, Lacan equates the source with the erogenous zones (also referred to as erotogenic zones by Freud).[35] Lacan asks:

> Why are the so-called erogenous zones recognized only in those points that are differentiated for us by their rim-like structure? Why does one speak of the mouth and not of the oesophagus or the stomach? They participate just as much in the oral function.[36]

Rather than answering this question directly he moves on to describe the drive in terms of a *montage*:

> The *montage* of the drive is a *montage* which, first, is presented as having neither head nor tail—in the sense in which one speaks of *montage* in a surrealist collage ... I think the resulting image would show the working of a dynamo connected to a gas-tap, a peacock's feather emerges, and tickles the belly of a pretty woman, who is just lying there looking beautiful.[37]

---

33 Dravers, 'The Drive as a fundamental Concept', 140.

34 Freud, 'Instincts and their Vicissitudes', 123.

35 However, Freud makes no mention of these in his paper. In fact, his only reference to 'erotogenic zones' is in his paper *On Narcissism*. (Sigmund Freud, 'On Narcissism: An Introduction', in *The Standard Edition of the Complete Psychological Works of Sigmund Freud* (London: Hogarth Press, 1914), XIV, 84.)

36 Lacan, *Seminar XI*, 168–169.

37 *Ibid.*, 169.

This is Lacan's rather colourful way of describing the 'deconstruction' of the drive into its four 'components' or 'elements (pressure, aim, object, source). Further on he argues that "The drive is precisely that *montage* by which sexuality participates in the psychical life..." which is linked to the structure of the unconscious.[38] Dravers remarks that the drive, as montage, is "...not organised to the end in view, but rather (is) susceptible to an almost infinite number of transformations and reversals."[39] In other words, the drive is not 'pre-programmed' to 'find' a particular object in order to gain 'satisfaction', for example in heterosexual relations. Rather, for each subject the drive has its own, unique trajectory. And with regards to the drive's 'almost infinite number of transformations and reversals' noted by Dravers, Lacan cites Freud's examples of the reversal of subject and object in the cases of sadism and masochism, and in scopophilia and exhibitionism.[40] He links this to a brief discussion of the 'grammatical' aspect of the drive:

> Incidentally, how can one say, just like that, as Freud goes on to do, that exhibitionism is the contrary of voyeurism, or that masochism is the contrary of sadism? He posits this simply for grammatical reasons, for reasons concerning the inversion of the subject and the object, as if the grammatical object and subject were real functions. It is easy to show that this is not the case, and we have only to refer to our structure of language for this deduction to become impossible.[41]

At the beginning of Lesson 14 of the Seminar Lacan argues that Freud's paper (*Instincts and their Vicissitudes*) falls into two parts: the deconstruction of the drive and a discussion of love.[42] He goes onto point out that

---

[38] *Ibid.*, 176.

[39] Dravers, 'The Drive as a Fundamental Concept', 133.

[40] Freud, 'Instincts and Their Vicissitudes', 127.

[41] Lacan, *Seminar XI*, 170. Although as Strachey notes (pp.127–128 of *Instincts and their Vicissitudes*), in this instance Freud is using the term 'subject' to mean 'agent', that is, the person who plays an active part in the relationship. Therefore, in the case where the 'reversal' is from sadism to masochism, the agent (Freud's 'subject) switches from one person to another, even though in grammatical terms the subject remains the same person.

[42] Specifically, this refers to pp. 133–140 of 'Instincts and their Vicissitudes'.

Freud is clear that love cannot be regarded as the sum of sexual feeling.[43] According to Lacan:

> The whole point of the article (*Instincts and their Vicissitudes*) is to show us that with regard to the biological finality of sexuality, namely, reproduction, the drives, as they present themselves in the process of psychical reality, are partial drives.[44]

This reiterates the point I made earlier that the drives are not 'pre-programmed' for heterosexual relations which aim at sexual reproduction.

Lacan then takes what appears to be a (quasi) biological turn by arguing that the drives are linked to an economic factor which "...depends on the conditions in which the function of the pleasure principle is exercised at a level that I will take up again ... in terms of the *Real-Ich*."[45] This *Real-Ich*, according to Lacan, can be conceptualised as the central nervous system which functions as a homeostatic system designed to regulate the internal tension of the drive. And he goes onto argue that "It is because of the reality of the homeostatic system that sexuality comes into play only in the form of partial drives."[46] This is important because it posits a relationship between drive regulation and the erotogenic zones, and in turn the impossibility of 'total satisfaction' of the drive. In other words, sexual pleasure is extremely limited, which is another way to define phallic jouissance, which will become especially important in Lacan's later work when he discusses the difference between phallic jouissance and the jouissance of the Other.

A key part of Lacan's 'deconstruction' of the drive is the idea of its *trajectory*, or its *circuit*, in which the drive emanates from the 'rim' of one of

---

[43] Freud writes:

> We should prefer to regard loving as the expression of the *whole* sexual current of feeling; but this idea does not clear up our difficulties, and we cannot see what meaning to attach to an opposite content of this current. (Freud, 'Instincts and their Vicissitudes', 133, italics in original)

[44] Lacan, *Seminar XI,* 175.

[45] *Ibid.*, 175.

[46] *Ibid.*, 176.

the erotogenic zones, then circles around the object *a* before returning to the rim. This is also a useful way to illustrate the repetition of the drive and the fact that the 'satisfaction' of the drive is precisely this endless circuit. Lacan plays on the two meanings of the French term *but* to differentiate between the aim and the goal of the drive. In doing so he employs the language of archery. He argues that the reason the drive can attain its satisfaction without reaching its biological aim (sexual reproduction) is because *but* can be seen as referring to the *trajectory* of the drive (as in the trajectory of an arrow), rather than something obtained. *But* can also mean *goal*, which in this case "…is not the bird you shoot, it is having scored a hit and thereby attained your *but*."[47] The rim refers to the source of the drive, that is, the erogenous zones. According to Lacan, this schema of the drive is a way to illustrate that:

> If the drive may be satisfied without attaining what, from the point of view of a biological totalization of function, would be the satisfaction of its end of reproduction, it is because it is a partial drive, and its aim is simply this return into circuit.[48]

Furthermore, in the process a new subject (*ein neues Subjekt*) "…which is properly the other, appears in so far as the drive has been able to show its circular course".[49] According to Dravers, what Lacan is saying here is that the schema of the drive not only shows its circular movement but also "…highlights the fact that this outward and backward movement necessarily presupposes a relation to the Other."[50]

The object *a* is what marks out the trajectory or orbit of the drive; in other words, the drive circles, endlessly, around the 'lost' object:

---

[47] *Ibid.*, 179.

[48] *Ibid.*, 179

[49] It is not clear from the text whether Lacan is referring to the Other, as in a structural position within language or the other, as in the specular other (person). Dravers in his commentary opts for the former meaning.

[50] Dravers, 'The Drive as a Fundamental Concept', 140.

> The *objet petit a* is not the origin of the oral drive. It is not introduced as the original food, it is introduced from the fact that no food will ever satisfy the oral drive, except by circumventing the eternally lacking object.[51]

Here Lacan is using the example of the oral drive (one of his four partial drives)[52] to illustrate the fact that the object *a* has nothing to do with an actual, material object, for example, food, which, once consumed, will 'satisfy' the subject. Rather, it is, paradoxically, the lack of (actual, material) satisfaction that 'satisfies' the drive. However, perhaps a rather more surprising example of the object *a* is that of the *gaze*, but in Seminar XI this features quite prominently. Lacan introduces this topic during his discussion of Freud's section on *Schaulust* (seeing and being seen) in *Instincts and their Vicissitudes*,[53] and argues that this is manifested in perversion—though the drive itself is not perverse:

> What constitutes the enigmatic character of Freud's presentation derives precisely from the fact that he wishes to give us a radical structure—in which the subject is not yet placed. On the contrary, what defines perversion is precisely the way in which the subject is placed in it.[54]

Lacan argues that in voyeurism the object is the *gaze* and he makes reference to Sartre's analysis of voyeurism in *Being and Nothingness*:

> The object, here, is the gaze—the gaze that is the subject, which obtains it, which hits the bull's eye in target shooting. I have only to remind you what I said of Sartre's analysis. Although this analysis brings out the agency of the gaze, it is not at the level of the other whose gaze surprises the subject looking through the keyhole. It is that the other surprises him, the subject, as entirely hidden gaze.[55]

---

[51] Lacan, *Seminar XI*, 180. In later texts, *object petit a* tends to be written as object *a*.

[52] The others being the anal, the scopic and the invocatory drives.

[53] Although it is not made clear in 'Instincts and their Vicissitudes', in his *Three Essays on Sexuality* Freud uses the term 'scopophilia' (*Schaulust*) to refer to *both* voyeurism *and* exhibitionism (see especially pp. 156–157), and this is what Lacan appears to be referring to in this section.

[54] Lacan, *Seminar XI*, 181–182.

[55] *Ibid.*, 182.

Antonio Quinet, in his text *The Gaze as an Object,* points out, the idea of the gaze as object can initially seem very strange. He goes onto explain that Lacan's reference to the gaze as object *a* comes from Merleau-Ponty's *The Visible and the Invisible*:

> Merleau-Ponty points to something that becomes central in Lacan's work: there is a preexisting gaze, a kind of staring at us by the outside world … For Merleau-Ponty there is an imaginary being behind the eternal gaze. Yet such a being doesn't exist. What exists is the split between what one sees and the gaze, a gaze which is neither apprehensible nor visible, a blind gaze which is erased from the world. It is exactly in this way that the drive manifests itself in the scopic order.[56]

This invisible gaze is the gaze of the Other, and as Quinet reminds us, although it may be invisible to the neurotic subject it is all too visible and present for the psychotic.[57] Lacan points out that the object 'appears' for the subject in the form of *shame*: the voyeur is suddenly made aware of the Other's gaze, for example, while he or she is peering through a keyhole at someone: "What he is trying to see, make no mistake, is the object as absence. What the voyeur is looking for and finds is merely a shadow, a shadow behind the curtain."[58] What's especially interesting here, perhaps, is the link that is being made between the object *a* and the Other, which I already hinted at earlier in Lacan's reference to the appearance of *ein neues Subjekt* in the circuit of the drive.

---

[56] Antonio Quinet, 'The Gaze as an Object', in *Reading Seminar XI: Lacan's Four Fundamental Concepts of Psychoanalysis*, ed. by Richard Feldstein, Bruce Fink, and Maire Jaanus (New York: State University of New York Press, 1995), 139–47.

[57] Quinet writes:

> How can we understand the gaze in the psychoanalytic sense? The most obvious place is to observe it is in psychosis where there is a failure of the gaze. For neurotics the gaze as an object has no consistency, no substance. It does not appear; it cannot be seen. But for the psychotics, the gaze can sometimes be felt and seen because the screen fails, which is another way of saying that the Oedipus complex fails. In psychosis there is something that shows the subject that the object is not lost. The gaze, then, which is absent for neurotics, is not lost for psychotics, a fact that becomes more evident if we consider the difference between the real and reality. (*Ibid.*, 145).

[58] Lacan, *Seminar* XI, 182.

As a way of concluding this section I would like to briefly touch upon Dan Collins' discussion of the drive (which he refers to as a 'debunking').[59] Collins is particularly concerned about the apparent ambiguity in Freud's writings regarding the drive and especially whether it should be regarded as a 'mental' or 'biological' entity. For example, with regards to the source of the drive he asks whether it is "…the organ stimulus, or is it the mental representation of that stimulus?"[60] This links back to my earlier remarks regarding the apparent 'duality' of the drive: as *both* idea *and* as biological process. Collins, however, does not accept this duality/ambiguity; for him "…the drive is entirely a mental construct. All the elements of the drive are mental."[61] By 'mental' Collins means rooted in signifiers and the signifying chain. In fact, he goes onto to argue that the drive should be thought of as a *code*. This relates directly back to my discussion in Chapter 3 regarding the regulatory function of language and its operation as a binary code. This is essentially at the level of the drive itself; in other words, the endless circuit of 1 s and 0 s corresponds precisely to endless circuit of the drive referred to above.

The idea of the drive being a 'mental' (psychical) entity also links closely to the concept of the *libido*, which Lacan will recast in terms of jouissance. Collins argues that contrary to many readings of Freud, libido should not be conceptualised in terms of energy—or, more precisely, not in terms of some crude form of bio-energetics; rather, libido is itself formed from a network of signifiers: "The libido is not just some vague energy but a signifying network that is established by the subject's history, by a dialectic of demand."[62] Again, at this point it is worth recalling my remarks in Chap. 3 regarding cybernetics: many of the concepts it utilises, for example, that of entropy, are taken from physics but are then reformulated for uses within the framework of information theory. Therefore, it is perhaps a bit misleading to argue, as Collins appears to, that libido is not energy but rather a signifying network. Instead, it might

[59] Dan Collins, "Debunking the Drive," in *Critical Essays on the Drive: Lacanian Theory and Practice*, ed. Dan Collins and Eve Watson, The Lines of the Symbolic in Psychoanalysis Series (Abingdon, Oxon: Routledge, 2024), 1–39.

[60] *Ibid.*, 9.

[61] *Ibid.*, 30.

[62] *Ibid.*, 24.

be better to argue that the energy of libido can be formulated *as* a network of signifiers. Furthermore, if jouissance is Lacan's way to conceptualise libido then it follows that jouissance itself can be formulated in terms of signifiers. And it is to his complex (and evolving) concept of jouissance that I will now turn.

Jouissance: Introductory Remarks

My aim in the previous section was to layout, in some detail, the fundamentals of Freud's theory of the drive and how it has been further developed by Lacan. In terms of my basic thesis this 'mapping-out' of drive theory is critical because, as I indicated in the introduction to the chapter, in my view the drive is the true 'foundation' of psychical trauma. However, in order to show how the drive 'produces' trauma it is now necessary to explore the relationship between the drive and jouissance.[63] This is because, as I will explain further, and following Freud's arguments in *Beyond the Pleasure Principle* (and, even more so in *Inhibitions, Symptoms and Anxiety*) the drive itself is a source of excitation which, in particular circumstances, can become overwhelming for the subject; in other words, they become *traumatised* by the effects of the drive. And another name for such effects is *jouissance*. However, before exploring the relationship between the drive and jouissance it is first necessary to explain what the term 'jouissance' itself means in Lacan's work.

To facilitate this discussion I will be using Jacques-Alain Miller's six paradigms of jouissance as a basic conceptual framework and making reference to other key authors where appropriate in order to clarify particular points in Miller's argument. In my discussion I will pass quite quickly over the first three paradigms because, in my view, it is only at the point of the fourth paradigm that Lacan's concept of jouissance starts to take shape in relation to the idea of drive-jouissance and its relation to trauma.

[63] Please note: in earlier Lacanian texts the term 'jouissance' has tended to be written in italics. However, more latterly the convention has been to write it without italics, and this is a convention I will follow in this work except where I am directly quoting from other texts who still use the italicised version.

Jouissance and Miller's Six Paradigms

As Miller points out, Lacan's theory of jouissance underwent a number of significant changes between the early 1950s and the late 1970s. Miller argues that this development of Lacan's ideas can be formulated as a series of *paradigms of jouissance*, six in all.[64] This approach to jouissance is useful for two reasons: firstly because it shows that jouissance was a concept, albeit evolving, that had been part of Lacan's work from very early on in his teaching; and, secondly, because it illustrates the way jouissance came to occupy a prominent position in the 'later' Lacan (broadly speaking from 1970 onwards), whereas before his work tended to be characterised by the prominence of language and the signifier. Or, perhaps a better way to put it is to say that the concepts of language and speech themselves underwent a transformation whereby speech is treated as jouissance and language is seen as a derivative of *lalangue* (see below).

Miller names the first paradigm the 'Imaginarisation of Jouissance', which refers to what he defines as the 'introductory' period of Lacan's work (up until the mid-1950s). The focus here is on *intersubjectivity* and its relation to *speech* and *language*:

> On the side of speech, Lacan readily develops intersubjectivity, ever subject to revision. On the side of language he stresses, ever more so, the autonomy of the symbolic, the fact that the signifying chain, as it runs in the Other, has its own requirements, a logic.[65]

It is perhaps interesting to note that in Lacan's early teaching (for example in *Seminars I* and *II*) the term 'jouissance' appears only very occasionally and is used to refer either to the subject's *enjoyment* or their *pleasure*.[66] Both terms are problematic because they tend to downplay the excessive and painful nature of jouissance, although in Lacan's later work 'pleasure' will become redefined as phallic jouissance.

---

[64] Jacques-Alain Miller, "Six Paradigms of Jouissance," *Psychoanalytical Notebooks*, no. 34 (December 2019): 11–77. (Hereafter *Six Paradigms*)

[65] *Ibid.*, 13.

[66] According to the Collins Robert French-English dictionary, the terms 'pleasure' and 'enjoyment' are synonymous when it comes to the English translation of jouissance.

Miller refers to jouissance in this period as an 'imaginary satisfaction' which comes from the ego, and to a tension between the 'autonomy of the Imaginary' and the domination of the Imaginary by the Symbolic. He then goes onto to argue that there is a progressive transposition of the Imaginary into the Symbolic, with the Imaginary providing material for the Symbolic.

The second paradigm he names the 'Significantisation of Jouissance', which refers to the period mid to late 1950s. During this period Lacan begins to detach the drives from jouissance, which at this point in his teaching is seen as Imaginary. Instead, the drives are structured in terms of language. Miller makes reference to *Seminar V (Formations of the Unconscious)* where Lacan introduces the term 'jouissance' in a formal way for the first time and states that jouissance should be seen as the opposite 'pole' to desire and the signifier.[67] Miller refers to Lacan's formula for fantasy $\$\lozenge a$: "...where the image in its signifying function is articulated to the symbolic function. This writing will remain for a very long time in Lacan's teaching as the symbol of the connection between the symbolic and the libidinal."[68]

According to Miller the significant point in the writing of this paradigm is, "...when the phallus, whose status as image already distinguishes it from the organ, is displaced in order to privilege its symbolic status".[69] And by the time of *Seminar VI* the libido itself becomes written into the signifier. Miller writes of the "effacement of jouissance by the signifier..." and of jouissance being absorbed into the symbolic.

The third paradigm is named by Miller 'Impossible Jouissance', and this is the time of *Seminar VII* (1959–1960). During this period jouissance is attributed to the Real—*das Ding* (the Thing). Miller makes reference to the *barrier* that the Real opposes to the Symbolic and the Imaginary. He argues that:

> This paradigm is no longer bound to a model of erasure of jouissance by the signifier which is open to an *Aufhebung* [to lift up], but to that of the

[67] Jacques Lacan, *The Seminar of Jacques Lacan Book V: Formations of the Unconscious* (Cambridge: Polity Press, 2017). (Hereafter *Seminar V*)

[68] Miller, *Six Paradigms*, 22.

[69] *Ibid.*, 22–23.

> vase, which Lacan borrows from Heidegger. The vase is a created object which is added to the world. It has at the same time, paradoxically, the property of introducing an absence, and in this way the possibility of filling it.[70]

Miller makes reference to Kant's moral law as being identical to *das Ding*—it has the "…same dumb, blind and absolute character."[71] There is an opposition between libido (jouissance) as desire, and libido as *das Ding*, as well as a clear opposition between pleasure and jouissance. Miller argues that the Thing is the Other of the Other, what is lacking in the Other. He also makes reference to going beyond the impasse of jouissance with the development of the objec*t a*:

> In one sense it is an impasse to isolate the Thing as beyond symbolisation … Lacan will put this impasse to work in the following seminars … by making jouissance, which emerges here under the forms of the Thing, beyond symbolisation, appear from now on as object. The development of the object a that follows is the precise response to this. There is no chance of forming a new alliance between jouissance and the Other if we don't go beyond the Thing as massive jouissance.[72]

There is one particular point arising in *Seminar VII* that deserves attention and this is the (apparently misleading) claim by Lacan that jouissance is the satisfaction of the drive. During a discussion of the death drive he states:

> The problem involved is that of *jouissance*, because *jouissance* presents itself as buried at the center of a field and has the characteristics of inaccessibility, obscurity and opacity; moreover, the field is surrounded by a barrier which makes access to it difficult for the subject to the point of inaccessibility, because *jouissance* appears not purely and simply as the satisfaction of a need but as the satisfaction of a drive—that term to be understood in the

[70] *Ibid.*, 28.

[71] *Ibid.*, 29.

[72] *Ibid.*, 32–33.

> context of the complex theory I have developed on this subject in this seminar.[73]

However, as Néstor Braunstein points out, Lacan goes onto argue that the concept of the drive is extremely complex and cannot be reduced to a theory of energetics.[74] The 'satisfaction' of the drive, it is important to reiterate, is precisely in its *failure* to obtain satisfaction, in the sense of 'finding' the lost object; rather the drive is 'satisfied' in its perpetual circuit around the object *a*:

> ...if we consider the drive in relation to the field of language and not a debatable biological or hedonistic transcription, we cannot accept the phrase "the satisfaction of a drive." This phrase is neither Lacanian nor Freudian because it confuses drive with necessity and the difference between these two registers has always been clear in our experience. If *jouissance* has to do with the drive it is insofar as the drive leaves a remainder of dissatisfaction that spurs repetition and, for that reason, the drive both historicizes and dissatisfies. We can also affirm that *jouissance* is the remainder of the drive's movement around the object because what is contoured is the void in the Thing, stumbling with the real, impossible to avoid.[75]

The fourth paradigm Miller names 'Normal Jouissance', which was developed during the time of *Seminar XI* (1964). Miller refers to "...an extraordinary antithesis between The Ethics of Psychoanalysis and The Four Fundamental Concepts of Psychoanalysis, in which Lacan poses a new alliance between the symbolic and jouissance."[76] Although I discussed Lacan's 'deconstruction' of the drive in *Seminar XI* at some length in the previous section, it is worth highlighting, through Miller's paradigm, where jouissance fits into this. In this paradigm, he argues, jouissance is achieved through the normal path of the drive, rather than being a transgression (as in paradigm 3). It is an 'automatic' jouissance which inserts itself into the functioning of the signifier and is linked to the

---

[73] Lacan, *Seminar VII*, 209.

[74] Néstor A. Braunstein, *Jouissance A Lacanian Concept* (New York: Sunny Press, 2020).

[75] *Ibid.*, 56.

[76] Miller, *Six Paradigms*, 33.

concepts of alienation and separation: "It is about showing that jouissance is not an addition in its own right, that it inserts itself into the functioning of the signifier, that it is connected to the signifier."[77]

Alienation unites identification and repression, whereby the subject exists as an empty set represented by a signifier. This is the division of the subject, but the signifier that represents the subject undergoes *repression.* Separation is a 're-translating' of the function of the drive and is a response to alienation (repression and identification). The unconscious is structured in the same way as the erogenous zones—as a pulsating ring. This is linked to the drive and the model of the vase which is filled with libido as the object (the myth of the *lamella*). Jouissance is formulated as a *mechanism* which is inscribed upon the functioning of a *system* "…instead of appearing irreducible to the symbolic, or instead of being entirely reduced to the signifier, jouissance is distinguished as such and at the same time inscribed upon the functioning of a system."[78]

The object *a* can be considered 'loose change' of the Thing: object *a* is jouissance, and is linked to the sexed body and its mortality, a loss of life:

> One can then introduce the objects of the drive as repairing and filling in this loss of life. Jouissance is therefore distributed in the development of Lacan's teaching under the figure of the *objet petit a*, that is, something more modest, scaled down, more easily handled than the Thing. The *objet petit a*, in Lacan, is the loose change of the Thing.[79]

The object *a* is an element of jouissance which is substantial (as in being a substance) and which is inscribed in the Symbolic but not as a signifier.

Pierre Skriabine, in his commentary on Lacan's approach to the drive in *Seminar XI*, argues that:

> …when Lacan reformulates this concept (the drive) on the basis of his elaboration of the object *a*, he displaces his emphasis from the drive's signi-

[77] *Ibid.*, 35.
[78] *Ibid.*, 40.
[79] *Ibid.*, 40–41.

> fying structure to its value as *jouissance*; this change can be seen especially in his topological elaboration of the drive in Seminar XI...[80]

Skriabine goes onto to argue that the purpose of the drive is satisfaction through the production of jouissance. More precisely, he states that the drive produces surplus-jouissance, which is the object *a*:

> The drive is satisfied in this looping itself; the object and goal are thus dissociated. Therefore the drive aims at and attains its silent satisfaction in a displacement of the very notion of the object and its function. At the beginning of its movement, there is the object *a*, the lost object, the fundamental cause, the structural support of the drive, the hole made in the Other. It is precisely, however, because the drive also brings the other and its jouissance into play, that it "is the only form of transgression that is permitted to the subject in relation to the pleasure principle". It is a forcing toward jouissance; there is a production, at its end, of a *plus-de jouir*.[81]

Although this may seem to contradict Braunstein's argument that I cited earlier, that is, that jouissance is *not* the satisfaction of the drive, the important point to emphasise here is that the drive's 'satisfaction' is obtained through its *circuit*, not through any 'attainment' of a particular goal. It is in this endless circulation that the drive 'produces' jouissance in the form of the object *a*. However, there appears to be another contradiction within Skriabine's argument: on the one hand he is arguing that the drive produces the object *a* in its endless circuit, and yet on the other hand the object *a* is what 'pulls' the drive around in its circuit. In other words, there seems to be a logical contradiction here because the object *a* cannot be both *cause* and *effect* of the drive's circuit. Perhaps one way to resolve this contradiction is to think of the object *a* as a *retroactive* cause of the drive. In other words, the object *a* only ever appears after the event (*nachträglich*) of the drive's circuit, even though it is in fact the cause of the drive's circuit in the first place. The retroactive character of

[80] Pierre Skriabine, 'Drive and Fantasy', *JCFAR*, 8 & 9, 1997, 28.

[81] *Ibid.*, 34. The quote in the penultimate sentence is from *Seminar XI*, p. 183. *Plus-de jouir* translates as 'surplus jouissance', which is a 'beyond' of phallic jouissance (see *Seminar XX*).

Nachträglichkeit is something I will be exploring in more detail in the next chapter.

The fifth paradigm, 'Discursive Jouissance', revolves around *Seminars XVI* (1968–69) and *XVII* (1969–1970) and *Radiophonie* (1970). The focus here shifts to the relationship signifier-jouissance as primal, with the signifier representing *jouissance* for another signifier (rather than the *subject*). The signifier is essentially *binary* (S_1 - S_2), which is linked to the concept of the *swarm*. This is because it is impossible to think of the isolated signifier or to establish it alone. Miller points out that in *Seminar XVII*:

> ...it is the signifying chain that Lacan presents as repetition or as knowledge. Signifying repetition had always previously been required by the subject for its signifying representation and by its division, which always leaves a part of the subject un-representable. All of *Seminar XVII* shows the repetition required by jouissance.[82]

The reference to repetition and knowledge is key here. In the third lesson of the Seminar Lacan argues that knowledge is a means of jouissance. This is developed out of his idea that jouissance is an effect of repetition; and what is being repeated, through the circulation of the drive, is what Lacan calls the *unary trait*. Lacan originally introduced the concept in *Seminar IX* and although the unary trait refers to the isolated signifier, he explains that he prefers the term 'unary' to 'single' (as in 'single signifier') because he sees the unary trait in terms of a *number*.[83] Raul Moncayo (who uses the term 'trace' instead of 'trait') explains that it is a term "...that Lacan borrowed from mathematics following Freud's use of the unary trait to explain a form of identification" and that "Once established, the unary trace becomes a system for non-diacritical marks that are not yet integers".[84] Such traces or traits are used to represent the concept of

[82] Miller, *Six Paradigms*, 55.

[83] Jacques Lacan, *The Seminar of Jacques Lacan Book IX 1961–62: Identification*, trans. Cormac Gallagher (Dublin: Unpublished translation by Cormac Gallagher, 2002). Lacan introduces the concept of the unary trait in lesson four of the Seminar (page 33 of the transcript).

[84] Raul Moncayo, *Lalangue, Sinthome, Jouissance, and Nomination* (Abingdon: Routledge, 2017), 6.

number and examples include tally marks and vertical bars which are repeated (for example, IIII represents the number four).

In *Seminar XVII* Lacan argues that knowledge "…is dominated, articulated by purely formal necessities, the necessities of writing, and in our day this leads to a certain type of logic." This 'certain type of logic', Lacan explains, is modern logic and although it might be regarded as the most 'purified' form of knowledge, it is the same knowledge that appears, in the guise of repetition, in the analyst's consulting room. Furthermore, according to Lacan:

> This knowledge here reveals it roots in the fact that in repetition, and in the form of the unary trait to begin with, it is found to be the means of *jouissance*—precisely insofar as *jouissance* goes beyond the limits imposed, under the term of pleasure, on the usual tensions of life.[85]

The essence of Lacan's argument here is that the signifier (the unary trait) is an *apparatus of jouissance*. However, there is a further key part of Lacan's argument, and this is that in its endless repetition, jouissance is *running down, disappearing*, which he refers to as its *entropy*. At the same time, though, something appears in place of this 'disappeared' or 'lost' jouissance, the object *a*:

> What becomes evident … is, as we were saying just before, that there is a loss of *jouissance*. And it is in the place of this loss introduced by repetition that we see the function of the lost object emerge, of what I am calling the *a*. What does this impose on us? If not this formula that at the most elementary level, that of the imposition of the unary trait, knowledge at work produces, let's say, an entropy.[86]

This 'lost object', the object *a*, is a 'stand-in' for the 'actual jouissance' of the subject, and in the same seminar is described by Lacan as *surplus jouissance*. However, in developing his concept of surplus jouissance Lacan also discounts his previous argument (in *Seminar VII*) that jouissance is a transgression, something forbidden; on the contrary, argues Lacan:

---

[85] Lacan, *Seminar XVII*, 48.

[86] *Ibid.*, 48.

> We are not dealing with a transgression, an irruption into some forbidden field through the wearing away of vital regulatory apparatuses (the pleasure principle). In fact, it is only through this effect of entropy, through this wasting, that *jouissance* acquires a status and shows itself. This is why I initially introduced it by the term "*Mehrlust*," surplus *jouissance* ... Only the dimension of entropy gives body to the fact that there is surplus *jouissance* there to be recovered.[87]

In other words, jouissance is an effect of the repetition of the signifier; a repetition that is 'powered' by the circuit of the drive. However, this is a jouissance that is perpetually 'decaying', so to speak, like the radioactive decay of certain particles. Or perhaps an even better analogy might be that of a collapsed star, where all that is left is a point of singularity (a black hole) around which all other stars (and other objects) circulate and, on occasion, are drawn too close to the event horizon of the collapsed object and disappear themselves. In the case of surplus jouissance and the object *a*, the 'star' in question is the subject's jouissance which has 'collapsed' to a point of singularity (the object *a*). Just as in astrophysics, where black holes are known by their effects on other objects, so in psychoanalysis the object *a* is known by its effects on the drive and the signifier, notably in repetition. And would it be stretching the analogy too far to suggest that trauma can be seen as the subject getting a bit too close to the 'event horizon' of the object *a*, whose overwhelming 'gravitational field' ('pull' on the subject) threatens to tear the subject apart?

According to Miller, this surplus jouissance can be regarded as a *supplement* to the loss of jouissance and as extending the register of the object *a* beyond 'natural' objects and encompassing those of industry and culture. These are the 'crumbs' of jouissance - 'minor *objet petit a*': "We see our cultural world inhabited by substitutes for jouissance, which are little nothings. These are crumbs of jouissance which give a particular style to our way of life and our way of enjoying."[88]

At this point it is important to note that Miller appears to contradict the idea that the object *a* is a 'product' of the drive, which was Lacan's

[87] *Ibid.*, 50.

[88] Miller, *Six Paradigms*, 61.

argument in *Seminar XI*. He argues that when jouissance "…is presented at the *objet petit a* of the drive, it belongs in a list …the oral object, the anal object, the scopic object, the vocal object…" These correspond to the partial drives that Lacan discusses in *Seminar XI*. However, Miller continues, "…when you think of jouissance as surplus jouissance, that is to say as that which fills in, but never exactly fills in, the loss of jouissance .. here the list of *objets petit a* increases and extends itself."[89]

What Miller is arguing here is that previously Lacan (following Freud) was arguing that the objects of the drive were all 'natural', that is, the erogenous zones of the body, and therefore the object *a* was related to the 'lost' jouissance associated with each of these zones. However, with the advent of the concept of surplus jouissance this effectively *generalises* the idea of jouissance; in other words, *anything*, any object in the world, can be seen as 'it', the source of the 'lost' jouissance. And clearly, this is what modern consumer capitalism plays on and exploits.

On the other hand, this does not negate the role of the drive in 'producing' surplus jouissance; rather, I would argue, it simply reiterates Lacan's argument, which I referred to earlier, that in the end there is only *one* drive, namely the *death* drive, which is the driving force of the repetition of the signifier. And Lacan is quite explicit about this in *Seminar XVII* when he states that "…the path towards death is nothing other than what is called jouissance."[90] This also links closely to the idea that the death drive is the 'motor force', so to speak, of the Symbolic order itself, which I discussed in the context of Lacan's 'cybernetic' concept of language.

Miller's reference to these 'crumbs of jouissance' (surplus jouissance) that can exist anywhere in the world raises an important question: if jouissance (in its 'supplementary' form) is 'out there in the world', so to speak, then was Freud right all along when he argued that trauma originates in external excitations that 'breach' the protective shield of the psychical apparatus? Or, to put it another way, where does jouissance come from in the first place? This is a question I will be addressing as part of the conclusion of this work, but for now I would like to move to explore

[89] *Ibid.*, 60.

[90] Lacan, *Seminar XVII*, 18.

Miller's sixth and final paradigm that he calls 'The Non-Rapport' and which is based around *Seminar XX* (1972–1973).

Before doing so, however, it is important to note that in this seminar Lacan argues that there are essentially two different modes: *phallic jouissance* and the *Other jouissance*, which in later seminars he also refers to as 'the jouissance of the Other'. With regards to phallic jouissance, which equates with the Freudian idea of pleasure, Lacan argues that:

> Analytic experience attests precisely to the fact that everything revolves around phallic jouissance, in that woman is defined by a position that I have indicated as "not whole" (*pas-tout*) with respect to phallic jouissance.
>
> I will go a little further. Phallic jouissance is the obstacle owing to which man does not come (*n'arrive pas*), I would say, to enjoy woman's body, precisely because what he enjoys is the jouissance of the organ.[91]

Lacan speaks of the two 'poles' of jouissance, one of which is phallic and the other is only glimpsed at:

> For one pole, jouissance is marked by the hole that leaves it no other path than that of phallic jouissance. For the other pole, can something be attained that would tell us how that which up until now has only been a fault (*faille*) or gap in jouissance could be realized?
>
> Oddly enough, that is what can only be suggested by very strange glimpses.[92]

Lacan also argues that "Jouissance, qua sexual, is phallic—in other words it is not related to the Other as such."[93] This is essentially the jouissance of the (sexual) organ; in other words, a very restricted and limited jouissance, the jouissance of (symbolic) castration.[94]

---

[91] Lacan, *Seminar XX*, 7.

[92] *Ibid.*, 8.

[93] *Ibid.*, 9.

[94] ...man is but a signifier because where he comes into play as a signifier, he comes in only *quoad castrationem*, in other words, insofar as he has a relation to phallic jouissance. (*Ibid.*, 35)

With regards to the jouissance of the Other, although the English title of *Seminar XX* is 'On Feminine Sexuality, the Limits of Love and Knowledge', the jouissance of the Other (or the Other jouissance) is not specifically related to women. Rather, it is a jouissance that transcends (or transgresses) phallic jouissance. In fact, one of the examples that Lacan uses in his seminar is that of the Christian mystics:

> Mysticism isn't everything that isn't politics. It is something serious, about which several people inform us—most often women, or bright people like Saint John of the Cross, because one is not obliged, when one is male, to situate oneself on the side of $\forall x \Phi x$. One can also situate oneself on the side of the not-whole. There are men who are just as good as women. It happens. And who also feel just fine about it. Despite—I won't say their phallus—despite what encumbers them that goes by that name, they get the idea or sense that there must be a jouissance that is beyond. Those are the ones we call mystics.[95]

The most famous example of such a 'mystical' jouissance given by Lacan in the seminar is that of Bernini's statue of Saint Teresa, whom many commentators have noted appears to be in a state of sexual rapture.

Miller's reading of *Seminar XX* is that it marks a return to *das Ding* through jouissance whilst at the same time "...pushing the indications of paradigm 5 to their conclusion." It also, according to Miller, marks a "kind of return to Peirce" because Lacan defines the signifier as a sign. Here, speech is treated as jouissance, and language and structure become a derivative of *lalangue*, "...which is speech before its grammatical and lexicographic ordering".[96]

Miller argues that in place of primordial/transcendental terms relating to *structure* there is the primacy of *practice*. This links to the idea that

---

[95] *Ibid.*, 76. $\forall x \Phi x$ is a way of stating that all men are submitted to the phallic function, that is, castration. It is one of the terms in Lacan's 'graph of sexuation' which is a way to 'map-out' the two 'modes' of jouissance discussed above. A full explanation of the graph can be found in lesson VII of *Seminar XX*.

[96] *Ibid.*, 64.

paradigm six can be represented by two Eulerian circles with the intersection marked as empty, which means there is a lack of connection between elements. Miller argues that this empty intersection is filled with *routine* (which can also be thought of in terms of *tradition*) and *invention*. This paradigm is the 'empire of the non-rapport' (as in 'there is no sexual rapport') which marks the demise of structuralism and "…in Lacan's final teaching, goes on to question the pertinence of trying to operate on jouissance on the basis of speech and meaning."[97] This is the point at which Lacan concludes that 'psychoanalysis does not work' in contrast to his original 1952 proposition that 'there is psychoanalysis'. However, there is jouissance, which is now seen as a property of the living body:

> All there is for psychoanalysis is a living body—one that speaks of course. Moreover, the 'and which speaks' [*et qui parle*] is again, for Lacan, in this seminar, something that must be described as a mystery … Put another way, the assumption is, 'through the body' [*par le corps*].[98]

Miller goes on to discuss the idea that 'non-rapport' "…makes the Other of the Other appear in the form of the One."[99] This means there is no (external) guarantee of the Other, only what he calls 'jouissance One' (or the One-jouissance), jouissance without the Other. He refers to contemporary individualism as being based on this concept of jouissance One:

> …which indeed renders problematic everything that is relationship and community, including even the marital bond, where even those whom we can call conservatives, those who sanctify routine as tradition, are irresistibly taken by the movement of invention, to establish through the means of positive law—as voted for in parliaments—relationships between individual atoms.[100]

With regards to the question of feminine jouissance, Miller, in another text, argues that feminine jouissance can be thought of in terms of

[97] *Ibid.*, 67.
[98] *Ibid.*, 69.
[99] *Ibid.*, 70.
[100] *Ibid.*, 71.

'jouissance as such', by which he means it is "...non-Oedipal *jouissance* conceived as subtracted from, outside of the Oedipus machinery. It is *jouissance* reduced to the bodily event."[101] And in his sixth paradigm, Miller stresses that all jouissance is jouissance of the body (jouissance One). *Phallic* jouissance can also be seen as a form of jouissance One which Lacan described as the jouissance of the idiot, "...of the solitary, a jouissance which is set up in the non-rapport to the Other."[102] Speech is jouissance, the *Blahblah,* which is the jouissance of the body. Miller concludes that the 'reign of the One-jouissance':

> ...renders the jouissance of the Other extremely problematic. Its very existence is cast in doubt. In any case, if it exists it is not on the same level as jouissance One. Jouissance One is real, whilst the jouissance of the Other now appears as a problematic construction.[103]

An Embodied Jouissance

Although I briefly alluded to it in the previous section, it is important to emphasise that in Lacan's later work the body, and more specifically, the jouissance of the body, moves centre stage; and in the process, I would argue, we see the emergence of what Miller has described as a 'Lacanian biology'.[104] Or perhaps it might be more accurate to speak of a *re-emergence* of such a 'biology', because, as I discussed in Chap. 3, it was already present in Lacan's second seminar. However, as Miller points out, in that seminar Lacan emphasised the fact that Freud's biology, being "first of all an energetics," is not biology. In other words, because Freud's concept of biology was heavily influenced by Fechner's psychophysics, it was not a biology as we would probably understand it, that is, as a science of life. But Miller goes onto argue that modern biology itself no longer

[101] Jacques-Alain Miller, 'Is Feminine Jouissance Not Jouissance as Such?', *Lacanian Lnk*, 55/56, 2021, 34–51, 37.

[102] Miller, *Six Paradigms*, 72.

[103] *Ibid.*, 75.

[104] Jacques-Alain Miller, "Lacanian Biology and the Event of the Body," *Lacanian Lnk*, no. 18 (2001): 6–29.

has life as its object. Instead, it is a … "biology without life, a biology which has as its object—this is one of Jacob's expressions, but it could just as well be Lacan's—'the algorithms of the living world'.[105] However, life reappears as the condition of jouissance; or, more precisely, the living body is the condition of jouissance. This is something Lacan makes clear in *Seminar XX*:

> Isn't that precisely what psychoanalytic experience presupposes?—the substance of the body, on the condition that it is defined only as that which enjoys itself (*se jouit*). That is, no doubt, a property of the living body, but we don't know what it means to be alive except for the following fact, that a body is something that enjoys itself (*cela se jouit*).[106]

It is important to note at this point that the body in question is not the Imaginary, 'whole' body that appears at the Mirror Stage; rather, it is the living body, but 'life' in this context is jouissance. In other words, to describe life as the condition of jouissance, as Miller does in his paper, seems to play on a double meaning: on the one hand there is no jouissance without the living body; and yet on the other hand, the condition of life itself is jouissance. However, there is another condition that Miller attaches to jouissance: that of the signifier:

> I can at once mention a second condition that adds to the condition of body so that something like the sufficient condition be attained. It is the signifier condition, if we settle for Lacan's formula that the signifier is cause of jouissance. Thus the perspective—life as condition of jouissance, the condition of body, the condition of signifier…[107]

The idea of the signifier as the cause of jouissance becomes clearer in another paper by Miller, *The Symptom and the Body Event*, where he also refers to trauma and the failure of the pleasure principle. Miller argues:

---

[105] *Ibid.*, 7.

[106] Lacan, *Seminar XX*, 23.

[107] *Ibid.*, 23.

> In traumatism in the Lacanian sense, the core of the traumatic event is not attributable to an accident. Or it is, but the possibility itself of the accident which leaves traces of affect on the full sense I've given, the possibility itself of the contingent accident, which is always necessarily produced, opens the incidence of language on the speaking being, and precisely on the body. The essential attachment is the tracing of language on the body … Lacan will condense this" … the signifier is the cause of *jouissance*, but this is written in the notion of the fundamental body event which is the incidence of language."[108]

The reference to Lacan is from *Seminar XX*:

> The signifier is the cause of jouissance. Without the signifier, how could we even approach that part of the body? Without the signifier, how could we center that something that is the material cause of jouissance? However fuzzy or confused it may be, it is a part of the body that is signified in this contribution (*apport*).[109]

Jouissance and Trauma

What though, has all this to do with *trauma*? My contention in this work is that trauma can be seen as an effect of the jouissance of the drive, in other words, the jouissance that is 'produced' by the endless circuit of the drive. In *Seminar XI* such jouissance was defined in terms of the object *a*, whilst by the time of *Seminar XVII* the object *a* itself becomes recast as surplus jouissance. Furthermore, in Lacan's 'Borromean formulation' in his *RSI* seminar[110] and his 1974 Rome lecture *The Third*,[111] surplus jouissance appears in the place of the knotting of the three rings (Real, Symbolic and Imaginary). Therefore, following the logic of my argument, this is also the place of trauma. Furthermore, in Lesson eight of *Seminar XXI* Lacan makes reference to a 'hole' in the Real and through

[108] Jacques-Alain Miller, "The Symptom and the Body Event," *Lacanian Lnk*, no. 19 (2001), 29.

[109] Lacan, *Seminar XX*, 24.

[110] Jacques Lacan, *The Seminar of Jacques Lacan Book XXII 1974–75: RSI*, trans. Cormac Gallagher (Dublin: Unpublished translation by Cormac Gallagher, 2011).

[111] Jacques Lacan, "The Third," *The Lacanian Review*, no. 7 (2019): 83–109.

the use of a neologism defines this as a *troumatisme*, which conveys the idea of the trauma as a hole or wound.[112] Braunstein uses this idea to convey the idea of jouissance as an "incoming excessive overload of excitations … impossible to control, that presents itself beyond the place of the Other, a muffled system of representations (Freud) or signifiers (Lacan)." He goes onto describe this jouissance as "ineffable, and illegal, traumatic … a hole (*trou-matisme*)" which "…marks the place of the impossible real."[113] Braunstein makes these remarks in the course of his discussion of Freud's idea of the traumatic memory. Referring to Freud's argument in the *Project* he writes:

> The patient who suffers from neurosis is a child who has passively lived a seduction perpetrated by an adult; sexuality first appears in the Other. That child has registered (in ω) the eruption of the external sexual real. The memory is a trace that cannot be integrated in the system of representations (or "neurons") that is the system of the ego (ψ) because its presence provokes an increase in tension that cannot find a pathway for discharge. In other words, the traumatic memory is a foreign body in relation to the ego that threatens the system as a whole. For the pleasure principle, which aspires to a balance of energy, this memory cannot be assimilated or accommodated and is thus separated from the recognized system of representations. In this way, memory becomes trauma, a wound and weapon that cannot be tolerated, the pain and suffering of an irreconcilable memory for the ego.[114]

The key point here is that the trauma is linked to the sexuality of the Other which manifests itself in the subject's ego as a memory that "cannot be assimilated or accommodated." Furthermore, the reason such a memory cannot be assimilated is because of the increase of tension (excitation) which Braunstein defines as "…a *jouissance* impossible to control,

---

[112] "But we all know, because all of us invent something to fill up the hole in the Real. Where there is no sexual relationship this gives a '*troumatisme*'" (Jacques Lacan, *The Seminar of Jacques Lacan : Book XXI : Les Non Dupres Errent: 1973–1974*, trans. by Cormac Gallagher (Dublin: Unpublished translation by Cormac Gallagher, 2010), 151. (Hereafter *Seminar XXI*)

[113] Braunstein, *Jouissance*, 23. Braunstein quotes Lacan as describing a 'hole in the symbolic' but in Lacan's seminar he refers to a hole in the *Real* (p. 151, Lesson eight).

[114] Braunstein, *Jouissance*, 21.

that presents itself beyond the place of the Other…"[115] The idea Braunstein wishes to emphasise is that jouissance "…thus comes to be the most exterior Other within oneself, a remembrance of the One that had to be renounced in order to enter the world of exchange and reciprocity. ."[116] The key point here is that the trauma of jouissance relates to both its 'externality' and its 'excess'. There are clearly strong echoes here with Freud's argument in *Beyond the Pleasure Principle*, where he defines trauma in terms of excitations that break through the protective shield which protects the 'living vesicle' (what Freud would later define as the *system Cs*).

But if Braunstein is arguing that trauma is the effect of the memory of the Other's jouissance in the subject, which 'Other' is he referring to? At first sight it might appear that he means the jouissance of the Other as in the jouissance of the body (referring back to Lacan's Borromean schema). On the other hand, it seems more likely that he is referring to a *specific other*, as in another person or subject, for example the mother, father or sibling. Strictly speaking, in Lacanian terms this would be the *specular other*, not the Other as a structural position and as a radical alterity.

In fact, there are strong echoes in Braunstein's analysis of trauma and jouissance with the work of Jean Laplanche, and especially his theory of childhood seduction which he lays out in *New Foundations for Psychoanalysis*. This is in spite of the fact that Braunstein never once references Laplanche in the 274 pages of his book and may well be a good example of the 'occlusion' of Laplanche's work in some Lacanian circles that I touched upon in the Introduction. The crux of Laplanche's argument is that childhood sexual experiences always involve another person, either an adult or an older child. Furthermore, and this is the critical point, the other person is also a sexual being who is experiencing enjoyment (*jouissance*) from the engagement with the child. This need not be sexual abuse; it could simply be a mother breast-feeding or cuddling her baby. The key point here is that the full meaning of the other person's jouissance and how it is being communicated to the infant child is lost on its recipient; in effect it gets 'lost in translation'.

[115] *Ibid.*, 23.

[116] Braunstein, *Jouissance*, 23,

This idea in turn resonates closely with Ferenczi's concept of 'Confusion of Tongues' as articulated in his paper of the same name.[117] In other words, the child is confronted with a language (a 'tongue') of sexual enjoyment and desire from the other person that he or she is unable to make sense of. In fact, Laplanche argues that Freud's theory of childhood seduction, 'abandoned' by him in 1897 (although as I argued in Chap. 2 the term 'abandonment' is a complete misnomer), needs to be reformulated as a 'general theory of seduction' which he outlines in *New Foundations for Psychoanalysis*. And essentially, this new theory is based on the idea of an enigma, for both child and adult (in fact, Laplanche refers to the 'enigmatic signifier), whereby neither child or adult recognise the adult's sexual desire and jouissance which is transmitted to the child in form of 'messages' which neither the child or the adult can properly decode.

But going back to the question of which 'Other' is Braunstein referring to when he speaks of the trauma of the Other's jouissance for the subject, I think there is a case to be made that it is *both* the other *and* the Other. Firstly, it certainly appears to be the case that he is referring to another human being, usually an adult and most often the mother (certainly this is Laplanche's argument). But, the (m)other's jouissance at question here is, in one sense, Other for both the mother and the subject. As Laplanche puts it, it is essentially an enigma that neither adult or child can make sense of. And as I discuss further in the next chapter, the enigma of the other's Other jouissance will continue to haunt the subject for the rest of their lives and is the basis of *Nachträglichkeit*.

Furthermore, although Braunstein refers to the subject's *memory* of the Other's jouissance, such a memory is constituted by signifiers. However, as Freud notes in the quote above, such 'traumatic memories' are, strictly speaking, memory *traces*, which are, in essence, isolated signifiers that escape meaning and have failed to be integrated into a signifying chain. And such isolated signifiers, which, it will be recalled, Lacan referred to as unary traits, are the effect of the drive's eternal circuit around the object *a* (surplus jouissance). It will also be recalled that in *Seminar XVII* Lacan

---

[117] Sándor Ferenczi, "Confusion of the Tongues Between the Adults and the Child (The Language of Tenderness and of Passion)," *Int. J. Psycho-Anal.* 30 (1949): 225–30.

referred to the unary trait as a form of knowledge (albeit very elementary) which is a means of jouissance; but a jouissance that is perpetually 'running down' and 'disappearing', leaving only surplus jouissance as a remainder (and reminder) of the lost Other jouissance.

So here we have in essence the concept of *drive-jouissance*; a term that Jean-Louis Gault's uses in his paper *Two Statuses of the Symptom*,[118] and one which Miller refers to in his paper Is *Feminine Jouissance not Jouissance as such?*[119] Gault argues that a neurotic "…is a subject who has found a solution to defend himself against the real. This solution relies on the Name-of-the-Father and the fundamental identification that goes with it." A defence against the Real is essentially a defence against trauma and, according to Gault "…always involves a repression of drive-jouissance." The problem here, however, is that such a solution always fails and the subject is "…contaminated by the return of drive-jouissance."[120] This suggests that even 'normal', that is, neurotic, subjects are beholden to the jouissance of the drive. And this is essentially the Lacanian thesis: we are all always already traumatised. The only question that remains, I would argue, *is where exactly is the trauma located?* It might be tempting at this point to refer back to Freud's theory of the traumatic neuroses and argue that such traumas are located in the 'outside world', but as I've already discussed, Freud also argued that the drive itself was a source of trauma. At the same time, though, Miller argues that the 'outside world' is now the source of many forms of surplus jouissance (his 'crumbs of jouissance') so perhaps things are not that simple; in other words, it is not simply a case of either the trauma is to be found in the external world or in the drive. However, before exploring this question in more detail, there is one other aspect or 'dimension' of trauma that I would like to explore (in the following chapter) and this is the rather peculiar idea of Nachträglichkeit and its relation to history and temporality.

---

[118] Jean-Louis Gault, 'Two Statuses of the Symptom: "Let Us Turn to Finn Again"', in *The Later Lacan: An Introduction*, ed. by Véronique Voruz and Bogdan Wolf (State of New York: Sunny Press, 2007), 73–82.

[119] Miller, "Is Feminine Jouissance Not Jouissance as Such?"

[120] Gault, Two Statuses of the Symptom', 80.

6

Trauma, *Nachträglichkeit*, Temporality and History

Introduction

In this chapter I want to explore, in some detail, what is probably the most peculiar aspect of trauma. One of its notable characteristics is that its symptoms often appear only after a substantial length of time following the 'original' experience. In fact, the onset of such symptoms can often be 'delayed' for years or even decades (and possibly centuries). And confronted by this 'delay' Freud developed his theory of *Nachträglichkeit*.[1] In this chapter I will begin with a discussion of Freud's basic theory and then explore how this has been taken up within the framework of French psychoanalysis, with a particular emphasis on Laplanche's concept of 'afterwardsness' and Lacan's use of the concept in the context of his theory of language and the drive. I will then explore the question of retroactivity in relation to *Nachträglichkeit* and trauma, and how this relates to wider questions of causality, temporality, and history. I will conclude by briefly discussing two examples of how these ideas have been taken up within a wider social context.

[1] Although there have been a number of attempts to translate the term *Nachträglichkeit*, some of which are discussed briefly in this chapter, in my view none of them are particularly helpful and I have therefore chosen to leave the word in its original German.

© The Author(s), under exclusive license to Springer Nature Switzerland AG 2025

L. Chapman, *Traumatic Neurosis Revisited*, The Palgrave Lacan Series,
https://doi.org/10.1007/978-3-031-89158-8_6

The concept of *Nachträglichkeit* is probably one of the most misunderstood of a long list of Freud's misunderstood concepts, not helped by Strachey's mistranslation of the German word as 'deferred action'. At the same time, I would argue that it is probably one of Freud's most radical ideas, and perhaps should be added to Lacan's list of fundamental concepts. What is particularly important about *Nachträglichkeit* is that it belies the commonly held notion that psychoanalysis is based on some form of 'linear determinism', in which the subject's history is determined by childhood experiences, and that psychopathology is rooted in childhood trauma. What *Nachträglichkeit* introduces is the idea that there is a *retroactive transcribing* of the original experience as 'traumatic' at a later date in the subject's history. And such a retroactive transcribing is linked closely to the operation of language and the drive.

The Basic Theory

Although Freud never devoted a whole paper to the idea of *Nachträglichkeit* it does appear throughout his work. It gets an early mention in his *Project for a scientific psychology*, where Freud cites the case of 'Emma', a young woman seen by him, who was unable to go into a shop alone. Freud linked this to a memory she produced in analysis of going into a shop at the age of twelve (Freud notes this was shortly after puberty) and being confronted by two shop assistants who were laughing together. At this point she ran out in fright. She then associated this incident with another memory when she was eight when she went into a shop to buy some sweets and the shopkeeper grabbed her genitals through her clothes. In spite of this experience, she went back a second time but stayed away thereafter. Freud argued that the laughter of the shop assistants provided the associative link with the original incident, which reminded her of the grin of the shop keeper as he assaulted her:

> The course of events can now be reconstructed as follows. In the shop the two assistants were laughing; this laughing aroused (unconsciously) the memory of the shopkeeper. Indeed, the situation had yet another similarity [to the earlier one]: she was once again in a shop alone. Together with the shopkeeper she remembered his grabbing through her clothes; but since then she had reached puberty. The memory aroused what it was certainly not able to at the time, a *sexual release*, which was transformed into anxiety. With this anxiety, she was afraid that the shop-assistants might repeat the assault, and she ran away.[2]

And in his letter (52) to Fliess, Freud writes:

> As you know, I am working on the assumption that our psychic mechanism has come into being by a process of stratification: the material present in the form of memory-traces being subjected from time to time to a *rearrangement* in accordance with fresh circumstances—to a *retranscription*. Thus what is essentially new about my theory is the thesis that memory is present not once but several times over, that it is laid down in various kinds of indications. I postulated a similar kind of rearrangement some time ago (*Aphasia*) for the paths leading from the periphery [of the body to the cortex]. I do not know how many of these registrations there are: at least three, probably more.[3]

However, it is perhaps in his commentary on the 'Wolf Man' case that Freud gives the most elaborate clinical example of *Nachträglichkeit*. Referring to his patient's famous 'wolf dream', which occurred when he was four years old, Freud writes in a footnote:

> At the age of one and a half the child receives an impression to which he is unable to react adequately (his parents copulating); he is only able to understand it and to be moved by it when the impression is revived in him at the age of four; and only twenty years later, during the analysis, is he able to grasp with his conscious mental processes what was then going on in him. The patient justifiably disregards the three periods of time, and puts his present ego into the situation which is so long past. And in this we fol-

[2] Freud, 'Project for a Scientific Psychology', 354, italics in original.

[3] Freud, *The Complete Letters*, 207, italics in original.

> low him, since with correct self-observation and interpretation the effect must be the same as though the distance between the second and third periods of time could be neglected. Moreover, we have no other means of describing the events of the second period.[4]

The key point here is that it reinforces the idea that *Nachträglichkeit* is not a 'delayed' reaction to an earlier traumatic event (which is implied by Strachey's mistranslation). In fact, the trauma does not even exist at the earlier point in time. Instead, it is only through a process of 're-transcription' that the trauma becomes constructed retroactively. Regarding the Wolf Man's dream at age four, which forms the cornerstone of Freud's analysis of the case, this is not technically a 're-transcription', but neither is it a 'memory', in the strict sense of the word, of a previous trauma (the Wolf Man witnessing his parents copulating when he was an infant). Instead, the dream appears to be a representation of the Wolf Man's anxiety. It was only twenty years or so later that he was able to 're-transcribe' such anxiety, to assimilate it into his subjectivity (with more than a little help from Freud).

Laplanche and *Nachträglichkeit*

As House and Slotnick have argued, it is the French psychoanalytic community that has kept *Nachträglichkeit* in circulation up until the present day.[5] Perhaps more problematic with the concept of *Nachträglichkeit* (which is usually translated in French as *après-coup*) is that there has always been an inherent tension, at least with regards to its various English translations, between the idea of it representing deferred action, or that of a 'ticking timebomb' waiting to 'explode' at a later date; and of it representing retrospective modification, in which later events revise the memory of earlier ones (this was Lacan's understanding of *Nachträglichkeit*).

---

[4] Sigmund Freud, 'From the History of an Infantile Neurosis', in *The Standard Edition of the Complete Psychological Works of Sigmund Freud* (London: Hogarth Press, 1918), XVII, 45, n. 1.

[5] Jonathan House and Julie Slotnick, "Apres-Coup in French Psychoanalysis: The Long Afterlife of Nachträglichkeit: The First Hundred Years, 1893 to 1993," *Psychoanalytic Review* 102, no. 5 (October 2015): 683–708.

And it is precisely this tension that Jean Laplanche explores in his approach to the concept of childhood seduction. Although I touched upon Laplanche's ideas in this regard in the previous chapter, I would now like to discuss them within the context of *Nachträglichkeit*.

The crux of Laplanche's argument is that childhood sexual experiences always involve another person, either an adult or an older child. Furthermore, and this is the critical point, the other person is also a sexual being who is experiencing enjoyment (in Lacanian parlance, *jouissance*) from the engagement with the child. This need not be sexual abuse; it could simply be a mother breast-feeding or cuddling her baby. The key point here is that the full meaning of the other person's jouissance and how it is being communicated to the infant child is lost on its recipient; in effect it gets 'lost in translation'. To quote Laplanche:

> "…après-coup" is a phenomenon that is not played out within the individual, within the intrapersonal, but rather within the interpersonal domain. Its specificity and its ability to reverse the "arrow of time" depends on this idea and this idea alone. In an individual, après-coup does not principally depend on the successive stages of the person's life. It depends, first of all, on the *simultaneous* presence of an adult and an *infans* (a preverbal child). The adult's enigmatic message (which itself is inhabited by the adult's own unconscious) constitutes the "avant-coup" of this process that introduces, within the receiver of the message, the *infans*, an initial disequilibrium. Then, in a second moment, in the après-coup, the enigmatic message drives the *infans* to translate, a translation which is necessarily imperfect. Such an avant-coup is characteristic of the earliest concrete, practical messages transmitted to the child by the adult in the unavoidable frame of the "fundamental anthropological situation".[6]

Laplanche argues that Freud's theory of childhood seduction needs to be reformulated as a 'general theory of seduction' which he outlines in detail in his book *New Foundations for Psychoanalysis*. And essentially, this new theory is based on the idea of an enigma, for both child and adult (in fact, Laplanche refers to the 'enigmatic signifier'), whereby neither child or

[6] Jean Laplanche, 'Problématiques VI: Après-Coup', trans. by Jonathan House and Thurston (The Unconscious in Translation, 2017), 167–168.

adult recognise the adult's sexual desire and jouissance which is transmitted to the child in form of 'messages' which neither the child nor the adult can properly decode.

Just to reiterate: this 'failure of translation' is what forms the basis of the trauma for the child, and is what continues to haunt them for the rest of their lives; and it is here that *Nachträglichkeit* enters the story. According to Laplanche:

> ...for the subject, the question [is] "what does he want from me?" [It] entails opening the whole retroactive movement of translation: a search for the secret of the enigmatic message which must always more or less escape his understanding. For the human being, for each of us, this is après-coup's bidirectional movement. The progressive movement, the movement forward in time, is that of the enigmatic message originally offered by the adult to the child as something "to be translated." The retroactive, backward movement is located in the succession of attempts at a translation of the message by the receiver, while recognizing that something of the enigmatic will be left out of every translation.[7]

In other words, at various points in their life, the subject will attempt to 'decode' or 'translate' the enigmatic (sexual) messages imparted to them by the adult 'perpetrator' in their childhood. However, such a 'translation' never completely succeeds and there is always a traumatic (Real) remainder or residue left. As a child the subject was unable to make sense of the message, to 'decode' or 'translate' it; and many years later, as adults themselves, they are still attempting to decipher the cryptic sexual messages from childhood, usually unsuccessfully. In fact, according to Laplanche, each failed attempt at deciphering or 'translation' is the essence of *Nachträglichkeit*. The subject may be able to make some sense of their memories of the experience, but something is always lost, something always escapes representation.

But what of Laplanche's reference, in the above quote, to a 'progressive movement forward in time' as a characteristic of *Nachträglichkeit*

[7] *Ibid.*, 167.

(*après-coup*)? This seems to suggest a much more 'deterministic' form of *Nachträglichkeit*, one that in the enigmatic 'original' message 'determines' the subject's later efforts to make sense of it. In fact, though, and as I pointed out earlier, there has always been an ambiguity with regards to the term *Nachträglichkeit* from the very beginning. On the one hand there is the concept of 'deferred action' (Strachey's preferred translation of *Nachträglichkeit*), in which the causal 'arrow of time' goes from past to future and which means 'past' events 'determine' 'future' ones. Laplanche, in his *Notes on Afterwardsness*,[8] argued that this in fact was Freud's view of *Nachträglichkeit*.[9] However, there is also the idea of 'retrospective-modification', in which later events revise the memory of early ones (what Laplanche refers to as the 'hermeneutic' conception of *Nachträglichkeit*).

Laplanche makes it clear he is not comfortable with this 'dichotomy' of meanings, that is, *Nachträglichkeit* as *either* 'deterministic' (the 'deferred action' model) *or* as 'retrospective-modification'. Rather, he attempts to combine both meanings; there is a real event (the childhood seduction) which 'determines' the subject's subsequent (and ultimately failed) efforts to make sense of such an event. However, these attempts at 'sense-making' involve retrospective or retroactive constructions, heavily influenced by events in the subject's present.

Lacan and *Nachträglichkeit*

A number of writers, for example, Haydée Faimberg,[10] have argued that it was Lacan who drew attention to the importance of *Nachträglichkeit* after a long period in which the concept had lain relatively dormant. In fact, Lacan himself makes this claim in his paper *Position of the Unconscious* where he states: "*Nachträglichkeit* (remember that I was the first to extract

[8] 'Afterwardsness' is Laplanche's English translation of *Nachträglichkeit*, but après-coup has tended to be used in the English literature instead.

[9] Jean Laplanche, 'Notes on Afterwardsness', in *Essays on Otherness*, ed. by John Fletcher, Warwick Studies in European Philosophy (London: Routledge, 1999), 260–65.

[10] Haydée Faimberg, "A Plea for a Broader Concept of Nachträglichkeit," *Psychoanal Q.* 76 (2007): 1221–40.

it from Freud's texts) or deferred action, [*après-coup*], by which trauma becomes involved in symptoms, reveals a temporal structure of a higher order."[11] Here, Lacan is discussing the 'closing' of the unconscious which, he argues:

> ...also demonstrates the core of a reversion time, quite necessarily introduced [if we are to explain] the efficiency of discourse. It is rather easily perceived in something I have been emphasizing for a long time: the retroactive effect of meaning in sentences, meaning requiring the last word of a sentence to be sealed [*se boucler*].[12]

What Lacan is getting at here is the idea that meaning is constructed retroactively and that it is only when someone has completed a sentence (for example) that its meaning becomes clear. This is something Lacan also emphasises in his initial discussions of the graph of desire in *Seminar V*.

And with reference to Freud's Wolf Man case he argues:

> Freud demands a total objectification of proof when it comes to dating the primal scene, but he simply presupposes all the resubjectivizations of the event that seem necessary to him to explain its effects at each turning point at which the subject restructures himself—that is, as many restructurings of the event as take place, as he puts it, *nachträglich*, after the fact.[13]

Here Lacan is emphasising Freud's point that *Nachträglichkeit* can be seen as a 'retranscription' of the memory of a previous event, which is effectively a *(re)construction*. Furthermore, as Freud pointed out, there can be *multiple* retranscriptions as the subject continues to try and 'make sense' of an experience which keeps evading sense. It is also important to note that although Freud focused on trauma as a retroactive construction, retroactivity itself is a characteristic of both language and the drive. This is

---

[11] Jacques Lacan, 'Position of the Unconscious', in *Écrits: The First Complete Edition in English*, trans. by Bruce Fink (New York: W.W.Norton and Company, 2006), 711.

[12] *Ibid.*, 711.

[13] Lacan, 'The Function and Field', 213.

something that becomes clear, for example, in Lacan's graph of desire, which he originally developed in *Seminar V*[14] and Seminar *VI*,[15] but which is probably better known for its inclusion in *Subversion of the Subject*.[16] As Lacan points out:

> …if I begin a sentence, you will not understand its meaning until I have got to the end. It's completely necessary—this is the definition of a sentence—that I say the final word for you to understand what the first was about. This provides us with the most tangible example of what can be called the *nachträglich* action of a signifier.[17]

Nachträglichkeit as Reverse Causality?

Earlier, I made reference to Laplanche's idea of the 'bidirectional movement' of *Nachträglichkeit* (après-coup), in the sense that the enigmatic message of the adult to the child takes place in a forward movement of time, whereas the subject's subsequent (and failed) attempts to 'translate' the message represents a retroactive or backward movement. This, however, touches upon a more fundamental question: to what extent does retroactivity represent some form of *reverse causality*? In other words, do events taking place in the present bring about something in the past? Going back to Freud's example of Emma that I discussed previously, when Emma went into the shop and encountered the laughing shop assistants this created an associative link with her previous encounter with the shop keeper who had assaulted her. And it was in the *present*, that is, in her encounter with the shop assistants, that she became traumatised. But the trauma itself was related to something that had happened previously, so is this an example of 'reverse causality'?

---

[14] Lacan, *The Seminar of Jacques Lacan Book V: Formations of the Unconscious*.

[15] Jacques Lacan, *Desire and Its Interpretation: The Seminar of Jacques Lacan Book VI* (Cambridge: Polity Press, 2019).

[16] Jacques Lacan, "The Subversion of the Subject and the Dialectic of Desire in the Freudian Unconscious," in *Ecrits: The First Complete Edition in English* (New York: W.W. Norton & Company, 2006), 671–702.

[17] Lacan, *Seminar V*, 9.

Or to give a more contemporary example, Bistoen, Vanheule, and Craps, in their paper on *Nachträglichkeit* and PTSD, elaborate the retroactive aspect of *Nachträglichkeit* in some detail in the context of post-traumatic stress disorder.[18] They cite the example of a young woman who had been raped (as an adult) but who did not in the aftermath of this experience exhibit any pathological symptoms. It was only when she heard that the same man had both raped and murdered another woman a few months later that she developed the symptoms of PTSD. As Bistoen et al. note, this puts a slightly different perspective on *Nachträglichkeit* to the one originally held by Freud, who argued that the phenomena tended to occur in puberty and 'triggered' a memory from an infantile experience. In this case the woman was already an adult when the 'original' experience occurred. Bistoen et al. argue that the woman may have been able to assimilate the attack on her, but the second attack (on another woman), which had resulted in murder, could have put her original attempts at interpretation, of trying to 'make sense' of that experience, into question.

And Bistoen et al. argue that Lacan's ideas regarding the signifier are especially instructive in terms of developing a deeper understanding of the mechanism of *Nachträglichkeit.* They argue that there is an 'original' distressing event that cannot be fully understood at the time of its occurrence because the subject is unable to symbolise it. However, the event leaves behind a 'mnemic trace' that is engraved in memory by a single signifier, which both signals and covers up the senselessness of the experience. Commenting on Freud's 'Emma' case, they write:

> This single signifier, which is metonymically chosen by the subject, hems in or borders the hole of the nonsensical experience. In Emma's case, this could be the linguistic element 'clothing' or the visual trace of the shopkeeper's grin, something that simultaneously points to and obscures the original mystifying scene. It is crucial to grasp that this single signifier or representation remains 'mute,' as it does not become associated with other elements that would confer meaning upon it.[19]

[18] Gregory Bistoen, Stijn Vanheule, and Stef Craps, "Nachträglichkeit: A Freudian Perspective on Delayed Traumatic Reactions," *Theory and Psychology*, 2014, 1–20.

[19] *Ibid.*, 9.

Their argument here is that it is only when this single signifier can form part of a signifying chain that it can allow the subject to confer meaning and 'sense' on their experiences. This happens at the time of the 'second' event where the subject realises, for the first time, the full meaning of the 'original' experience, and at this point becomes traumatised by it. Going back to their example of the woman who has been raped, the logic here is that she hears about another woman who has been raped and murdered by the same man and this in turn 'constructs' the trauma of an earlier event, that is, the woman's own experience of being raped. Now clearly the earlier assault of the woman is not 'brought about' by her hearing about the subsequent attack on the other woman; however, according to the theory of *Nachträglichkeit*, what is 'brought about', that is, constructed, is the *trauma of her own experience.*

It should be said at this point that not all writers subscribe to the idea of *Nachträglichkeit* involving some form of 'reverse causality'. For example, Thomä and Cheshire are very critical of the idea of 'retroactive causation' and point out that there is nothing in the concept of *Nachträglichkeit* that requires a reversal of the 'arrow of time'. They argue that:

> ...there is ... a needless muddle between (a) the logical 'direction' (so to speak) of the inference being made by the analyst or theorist who postulates *Nachträglichkeit* in a particular case, (b) the direction of the causal relationships which are being proposed by such an inference, and (c) the direction of the reconstrual or meaning-attribution being made by the person in question. Of course, both the therapist's inference and the subject's reconstrual are somehow backward-directed: but it does not follow from this that the *causal mechanisms* which are postulated as obtaining between the various events and experiences are themselves backward-directed.[20]

They go onto argue that the (temporal) orientation of *Nachträglichkeit* is only *metaphorically* retroactive, and not *actually* reversing the flow of time. But even if this is true, in the context of *Nachträglichkeit* what does

[20] Helmut Thomä and Neil Cheshire, 'Freud's Nachträglichkeit and Strachey's "Deferred Action": Trauma, Constructions and the Direction of Causality', *Int. R. Psycho-Anal.*, 18 (1991), 413, italics in original.

it mean to speak of retroactive causation, that is, the idea that effect precedes cause? Or, to put it another way, what is the *effect* and what is the *cause* in this case?

One of the (savage) ironies of *Nachträglichkeit* is that it is only when the subject is psychically developed enough to 'process' the original experience that they experience trauma. And such 'processing' often only occurs when, at time T_2, the subject has another experience which triggers a temporal 'looping-back' to the first experience at T_1. But it is not a matter of the second experience 'reminding' the subject of the first one and how traumatic it was; rather, the second experience *constructs* the traumatic memory of the first one. But is it accurate to argue that this is in fact a case of retroactive causation? For this to be the case the event at T_2 has to *cause* the event at $T_{1.}$ As I indicated earlier, writers such as Thomä and Cheshire would argue that this is *not* what happens. Making reference to Freud's own thoughts on *Nachträglichkeit*, they argue that he:

> ...makes it clear that what is doing the 'causing' in the here-and-now state of the psychic apparatus (the dynamic system in question) is the memory-*trace* of the original traumatic experience (E1), and not the original experience itself. Thus the causal action, or some part of the causal potential, of the original experience has indeed been 'deferred' from T1 to T2, (or even to Tn) but takes effect eventually, in combination with the effects of some critical later event (E2), through the medium of the memory-trace which is then (at T2) co-present in the dynamic system with its causal effect.[21]

They go on to argue that:

> It is beside the point, for the moment, that such access to the objective nature of the historical E1 (the 'original' trauma) may be therapeutically irrelevant, as Kris and others have been arguing influentially for some time ... However, it is important to emphasize that, even in this sense of *a posteriori* reconstrual, the orientation of *Nachträglichkeit* is only *metaphorically* 'retrospective', since no process (whether causal or psychological) is actually working backwards in time, as is suggested by phrases like 'retrogressive movement of psychic material', 'retroactive' and 'regressive movements'.[22]

---

[21] *Ibid.*, 414–415, italics in original.

[22] *Ibid.*, 415, italics in original.

But what 'category' of time are they referring to when they argue that there is no 'actual' reversal of time, that is, of causality? Their basic argument is that it is the *memory* (trace) of the 'original' event that is causing the trauma in the here-and-now, not the *actual* event itself. And the importance of the memory trace is something that Bistoen et al. emphasise in their paper, although they prefer the term 'mnemic trace' instead. They argue that such a mnemic trace is the equivalent of a single signifier and in relation to the first or 'original' experience:

> ...the first experience is retained in a very specific way: as a single signifier that borders the nonsensical event and that is unable to articulate itself with the rest of the psychic material. It is not accessible for conscious recollection, as it cannot be brought into articulation with the group of signifiers (or representations) that constitutes the Ego...[23]

However, at a later date the subject has another experience:

> ...which results in the *realization* of the first scene—realization, in the sense that the new experience gives birth to an understanding of what the subject had missed in the first experience. But more essentially: through this understanding, it is as if the potentially traumatic aspects of the scene that were not experienced at T1 (the time of the first experience) are now fully experienced at T2. The subject, through T2, receives access to the traumatic truth of the T1 event *for the very first time*. The T1 experience starts to be lived as a new subjective event.[24]

It is important to note the phrase 'as if' in the above quote; the authors seem to be suggesting that there is something metaphorical (to use Thomä and Cheshire's term) about the process. However, this raises the question as to whether Bistoen et al. are arguing that at time T1 there is no actual trauma or not. Clearly, *something* happens to the subject (and on this point Thomä and Cheshire are in agreement), but the key point here is that this 'something' is only *registered* by the subject as 'traumatic' at a later date. At the same time, though, Bistoen et al. are arguing that the

[23] Bistoen et al., '*Nachträglichkeit*', 10, italics in original.

[24] *Ibid.*, 10, italics in original.

'original' experience leaves a mnemic trace in the form of a single signifier, which forms the nucleus of the later 'realisation' (symbolisation) of the experience as traumatic.

But is *remembering* the same as *causation*? One of the problems with memory, as Freud himself noted and as psychologists and neuroscientists have argued ever since, is that it undergoes continuous *reconstruction*; in other words, what is remembered is not a naïve representation of 'what actually happened'. Rather, what is remembered is being continually reworked (or, to use Freud's term, 're-transcribed') which means there can be no such thing as an 'original' or 'authentic' memory of a particular event. And, of course, such a reworking or retranscription is taking place in the here-and-now, in the present, which seems to suggest that the present is impacting on the past, albeit in the form of *representations* of events in the past. But at the end of the day, such representations are all we have to go on, so in this sense, *and this sense only*, it would appear that the present *can* change the past, and therefore it is correct to argue that *Nachträglichkeit* is indeed an example of retroactive causation.

Or is it? If we go back to Bistoen et al.'s argument and their idea of a mnemic trace, then this suggests that even if the subsequent reconstruction (in memory) of the 'original' event is precisely that, that is, a reconstruction, there is still something remaining outside of the representation of the event. And this something, this remainder, this memory trace, is the Real. If this is the case then it would seem the trauma was there all the time, in the form of the mnemic trace, the single signifier. However, this is not the same as arguing that the subject was *traumatised* by such a trauma at the time of its occurrence.

But what of Laplanche's concept of the 'bidirectional' nature of *Nachträglichkeit*? Although it is not altogether clear whether he subscribes to the idea of 'reverse causality' or not, he certainly seems to be subscribing to the idea of time moving in two different directions. But in my view Laplanche appears to be making a fundamental error. He refers to the idea of the adult (the other) giving enigmatic messages to the infant subject and that this is taking place in 'chronological' time, that is, in a temporal movement from 'past' to 'future'. *But this is a retroactive construction by Laplanche himself.* In other words, he is creating a historical narrative of the encounter between adult and infant subject in order for his theory of childhood seduction to 'work'. This is *not* to say such an encounter never happened—far from it. Rather, it is simply to point out that it is virtually impossible to give an accurate account, historically (retroactively) of what actually happened. So in fact, there is nothing 'bidirectional' about Laplanche's theory of *Nachträglichkeit*; rather, the whole theory relies on the notion of retroactive construction. At the same time, though, this does not imply that retroactive construction represents 'reverse causality'. Rather, it means that such a construction is itself taking place in a 'forward' temporal movement; in other words, the 'arrow of time' only goes in one direction—from past to future.

And, perhaps more critically, it raises the whole question of what *temporal status* to grant to retroactive trauma; in other words, if a subject starts to experience traumatic symptoms years, or even decades, after a particular event, then *when* can the trauma be said to have occurred? According to the theory of *Nachträglichkeit*, the answer is in the *present*; or, to be more precise, whenever the event that led to the construction of the traumatic memory occurred. However, this raises an even more fundamental question: to what extent is the mnemic trace of the 'original' traumatic event, even 'within' time at all? Or, to put it another way, to what extent does trauma represent a completely different temporal order or category?

Nachträglichkeit, Trauma and History

One way to approach this question is to explore how *Nachträglichkeit* relates to the concept of *history*. More precisely, to what extent does *Nachträglichkeit construct* history—both at the level of the individual human subject and at the collective or cultural level? The key point to remember here is that history is essentially a 'function' of the Symbolic register; in other words, history is only possible within the framework of language and discourse, that is, within the network of signifiers.

In order to illustrate this I will now turn to Jacques-Alain Miller's paper *The Space of a Hallucination*, in which he develops Lacan's idea of *hystory* in order to show how history is only possible within the order of language.[25] He borrows the term from Lacan's *Preface to the English Edition of Seminar XI*, in which Lacan makes a play on the words 'history' and 'hysteria':

> Now, somewhat belatedly, I add my two cents' worth: a fact of hystory, let's just say hysteria—that of my colleagues, as it happens, a case of minor importance, but one in which I happened to find myself implicated for having taken an interest in someone—the Aimée of my thesis—who led me to drift over to them through having foisted Freud on myself.[26]

Rather than analysing the whole of this rather opaque paragraph, Miller picks up on the single line 'a fact of hystory, let's just say hysteria'. In the following quote, the two texts referred to are the *Preface* already mentioned and Lacan's *Response to Jean Hyppolite's Commentary on Freud's 'Verneinung'*: [27]

> From what I expounded to you last time, I will retain this opposition between the two terms "history" and "real" that I found at work in these two texts. What the later text adds is that with respect to the real, history is hystory, that is, hysteria.
> history and the real
> hystory
> hysteria
> This short-circuit is warranted by the "Preface," where one finds the following: "a fact of hystory, let's just say hysteria." History with an "i," hystory with a "y" and hysteria are, then, placed in a series. This witticism has to be given its full weight insofar as hysteria constitutes a psychopathological structure in which the impact of the Other, its discourse and its desire, on the subject is displayed in its purest from. This brings us to the angle from which Lacan first approached Freud's teaching, namely the definition of the unconscious as the discourse of the Other.[28]

---

[25] Jacques-Alain Miller, "The Space of a Hallucination," *The Lacanian Review* 6, no. 6 (2018): 82–107.

[26] Jacques Lacan, "Preface to the English Edition of Seminar XI," *The Lacanian Review*, no. 6 (2018): 22–27.

[27] Jacques Lacan, 'Response to Jean Hyppolite's Commentary on Freud's "Verneinung"', in *Écrits The First Complete Edition in Englsih*, trans. by Bruce Fink (New York: W.W. Norton & Company 2006), 318–33.

[28] Miller, 'Space of a Hallucination', 83–85. Please note: this was published in bi-lingual form, hence the page range.

Miller is drawing on the first part of Lacan's 'Rome Report', where Lacan argues that the unconscious is the subject's history:

> What we teach the subject to recognize as his unconscious is his history—in other words, we help him complete the current historicization of the facts that have already determined a certain number of the historical "turning points" in his existence. But if they have played this role, it is already as historical facts, that is, as recognized in a certain sense or censored in a certain order.[29]

One of key points about Lacan's argument in this section, and something which is emphasised by Miller as part of his wider thesis, is that the subject's historicisation effectively occludes the Real, and the Real of the subject's trauma. This is made especially clear in the following quote from Lacan:

> For to say of psychoanalysis and of history that, qua sciences, they are both sciences of the particular, does not mean that the facts they deal with are purely accidental or even factitious, or that their ultimate value comes down to the brute aspect of trauma.
>
> Events are engendered in a primal historicization—in other words, history is already being made on the stage where it will be played out once it has been written down, both in one's heart of hearts and outside.[30]

According to Miller, this represents the "supremacy of the true over the real." And insofar as 'truth', at least during this period of Lacan's work (the early 1950s), is within the realm of the Symbolic order, then the Real (and trauma as a manifestation of the Real) is repressed.[31] As Miller puts it: '…in Lacan's first advances, the concept of trauma disappears because historicization is primary. A trauma is already a "historical stigma"'.[32] In other words, trauma is always already situated within the Symbolic order, the domain of narrativisation and meaning.

---

[29] Lacan, 'The Function and Field', 217.

[30] *Ibid.*, 216.

[31] For a discussion regarding Lacan's different conceptions of 'truth' see D. Evans, *An Introductory Dictionary of Lacanian Psychoanalysis* (London: Routledge, 1996), pp. 215–17.

[32] Miller, 'Space of a Hallucination', 89–91.

And this seems to chime with the idea of *Nachträglichkeit* as retroactive construction; the subject only becomes traumatised 'after the event' and as a result of a temporal 'looping back' from a later to an earlier moment in time. It also rules out the idea of an 'original trauma', at least in the sense of the subject being traumatised at the time of the earlier event or experience. However, it should be emphasised that the idea of 'earlier' and 'later' moments in time, and, along with it, the concept of 'original trauma', is already to place us within the realm of history and narrative. In other words, there can only be an 'origin' within a symbolic framework, and along with it, the whole concept of 'past', 'present' and 'future'. So perhaps it might be more helpful to argue that within the framework of *Nachträglichkeit* the trauma always comes 'later' or 'afterwards', which strictly speaking is not the same as there not being an 'original' trauma. Or, to put it another way, within this framework, the idea of an 'origin' has a different meaning to that of an *actual* 'original' trauma. In Lacanian terms, an 'origin' is essentially the signifier S_1 which acts as an 'anchoring point' for a chain of signifiers $S_1 \ldots S_n$ which is what creates the chain of signification that constitutes the narrative of history. An actual 'original' trauma, on the other hand, equates far more closely with the isolated signifier itself.

And this brings me onto a broader question. Up until now I have been looking at the concept of history and *Nachträglichkeit* in relation to hysteria (the idea of 'hystory'). This might suggest that both history and *Nachträglichkeit* are 'functions' of hysteria, or more broadly, neurosis. In other words, history and *Nachträglichkeit* are dependent on a particular clinical structure which is characterised by a particular form of negation, that is, *repression*. Although, as House and Slotnick point out in their review of *Nachträglichkeit* in French psychoanalysis, Lacan appeared to first emphasise the concept in relation to *psychosis*, they also note that his use of the term (which he translated as *après-coup*), only appears once in that context.[33] Therefore, I would argue, this is hardly a basis for arguing that *Nachträglichkeit* can be used within the framework of psychosis and foreclosure. However, with regards to the question of history itself, it

[33] This is in the context of Lacan's commentary on the 'Wolf-Man' case in his 'Rome Report'.

would seem to become problematic once we move beyond the realms of the Symbolic order, which is also the domain of neurosis.

Going back to Miller's paper, *The Space of a Hallucination*, having explored Lacan's notion of hystory and the privileging of truth (the Symbolic history) over the Real, he goes onto argue that in Lacan's later teaching his theory of the unconscious shifts from being based on history and hysteria to being based on psychosis. And he develops this argument in the context of Lacan's response to Jean Hyppolite's commentary of Freud's *Verneinung* paper, which I referenced earlier, and especially Lacan's remarks concerning the Wolf Man case:

> Prior to his constructions of the history-unconscious, he [Lacan] had … entered Freud's theory from the angle of psychosis. This is also what justifies me in seeking the blueprint of his final text in his commentary on Freud's "*Verneinung*," the hallucination of the Wolf Man's severed finger. In the way Lacan approaches this hallucination, it calls the primacy of historicization into question. He presents it as a phenomenon that escapes history as well as the subjective and semantic reworking of truth. For an element to be historicized, and it is in this respect that Lacan goes further than his "Rome Report," it has to have been symbolized. There can only be a primary historicization if there is a primary symbolization.[34]

In other words, as I argued at the beginning of this section, for history to be possible there has to be symbolisation, that is, the Symbolic order itself has to be operating, which is not the case in psychosis. But where does that leave us with regards to *trauma*? Is this not also a 'failure' of symbolisation? To the extent that trauma can be seen as a manifestation of the Real (Lacan's argument in *Seminar XI*) this certainly seems to be the case, which also means that history (Miller's 'hystory') and trauma are incompatible. This in turn seems to suggest that trauma 'occupies' a different order of temporality which cannot be historicised.

Perhaps, then, we can even begin to think about two different orders of time: *historical* time and *trauma* time. If this is the case then what exactly is the function of *Nachträglichkeit*? If, following Freud's argument, the process of *Nachträglichkeit* retroactively constructs a trauma then

[34] *Ibid.*, 93

there seems to be an inbuilt contradiction because the concept of construction implies the operation of language. Indeed, as Freud argues in his paper *Constructions in Analysis*, constructions play a key role in psychoanalysis, especially when the subject fails to remember key events in their history.[35] To put it another way, how can a symbolic operation, which is what *Nachträglichkeit* is, *construct* something 'beyond' the Symbolic order? It seems more reasonable to argue, perhaps, that in spite of its best efforts, *Nachträglichkeit* represents a *failure* to (completely) symbolise trauma. This fits in well with Freud's idea of *Nachträglichkeit* as a series of retranscriptions (which are never quite completed) and Laplanche's idea of *Nachträglichkeit* as a series of (failed) translations as the subject struggles to make sense of the Other's jouissance.

Nachträglichkeit and the Failure of Historicisation

At this point I would like to pull all the strands of my argument relating to *Nachträglichkeit* together and propose the following thesis. *Nachträglichkeit* is the psychical process by which the subject attempts to signify or historicise certain experiences which they struggle to make sense of. Such experiences, following Laplanche, can be described as *enigmatic*. Furthermore, the very process of historicisation constructs the idea of such experiences as having occurred 'in the past', and often in early childhood. However, such a 'psychical' history has very little to do with the subject's *chronological* history. What such a history does do, however, is to construct a *narrative* or *story* of trauma, which, to a certain extent at least, does 'make sense' to the subject. This process of historicisation or narrativisation may continue for many years or even for a lifetime, for example in therapy, in support groups, in written histories, and so on. The subject experiences trauma to the extent that they cannot fully 'make sense' or give meaning to such an enigma, and the subject may spend the

[35] Sigmund Freud, "Constructions in Analysis," in *The Standard Edition of the Complete Psychological Works of Sigmund Freud*, vol. XXIII (London: Hogarth Press, 1937), 255–70.

rest of their life struggling to find meaning to the enigma. In other words, trauma represents a failure of historicisation.

The retroactive nature of *Nachträglichkeit* is one of its most striking and peculiar characteristics but is also one that is subject to a great deal of misunderstanding. In one sense retroactivity is simply a characteristic of language itself, insofar that meaning is only ever constructed after the event (*nachträglich*). However, retroactivity is also a way to describe the movement of the drive, which is constantly orbiting around the object *a* and producing jouissance. This suggests that there are two dimensions of retroactivity: firstly, the dimension of signification, that is, the construction of meaning, which is part of the process of regulating jouissance through the operation of the pleasure principle, that is, language; secondly, the retroactive movement of the drive, which is perpetually generating jouissance and, potentially, trauma in form of excess excitation. Strictly speaking, I would argue, *Nachträglichkeit* applies to the first dimension but not the second. To reiterate, in my view *Nachträglichkeit* does not *construct* trauma; rather, it is a failed attempt to 'de-traumatise' trauma.

Trauma Time and *Nachträglichkeit* as History

I would like to end this chapter by briefly exploring two aspects of trauma within a wider social context. So far in this work I have concentrated on trauma as an *intrasubjective* phenomenon, that is, how it is constructed and sustained within individual human subjects. However, I think it is important to remember that trauma never takes place in a social vacuum; in fact, there is a social dimension 'built into' trauma from the very beginning of foundation of the subject. This is the subject's relation to, and, reliance upon, the Other, and, more especially, the Other's desire and the Other's jouissance, although this is with the caveat that the concept of the Other, according to Miller, is a problematic one.

One of the dimensions of trauma I would now like to discuss briefly is the idea of *trauma time*; in other words, the idea I touched upon earlier that trauma 'resides' in a different order of temporality—or perhaps, it might even be better to argue that trauma is *atemporal*. In his essay

Memory's Time: Chronology and Duration in Holocaust Testimonies, Lawrence Langer makes a distinction between "chronological" and "durational" time.[36] Chronological time presumes a "before, during, and after", whereas in durational time there is only "now", and therefore there can be no sense of "what next?" or an "afterwards". Langer's argument is that for Holocaust survivors, time was durational rather than chronological, even when decades later they were giving their testimonies. Langer cites Lyotard's comment that Holocaust time is 'lost time', which has no place in the psychical apparatus, and points out that Holocaust time is a constantly re-experienced time. This means that it makes no real sense to talk about "Holocaust memory", because nothing is remembered; rather, it is repeated.

Another important point that Langer highlights is the importance for many Holocaust survivors—and the broader culture within which they are situated—of giving a meaning to their experiences. This applies particularly to the deaths of the victims, and, to use Langer's terminology, has given rise to the idea of the "Auschwitz death" as "sacrifice" or "martyrdom". The reality, however, as Langer points out, was very different:

> The idea of a "beautiful death" invoked by words like "sacrifice" and "martyrdom" awakens the consolations of chronological time, but the price one pays is fidelity to the durational moment: that is, the last gasp of life, followed by the literal annihilation of the remains, until no trace is left, in memory or fact, of what was once a human being. The language of chronology seeks to rescue the victim from that mute fate.[37]

In other words, the concept of a "beautiful death" invokes the idea of a meaningful death, which brings us back, paradoxically perhaps, into the land of the living: the world of "normal", chronological time, of "history" as most people understand it. Langer also briefly touches upon another aspect of "Holocaust time": he refers to the Auschwitz experience as a *splitting*, rather than a *continuity*, of time. However, we need to think of

[36] Lawrence L. Langer, 'Memory's Time: Chronology and Duration in Holocaust Testimonies', in *Admitting the Holocaust: Collected Essays* (New York: Oxford University Press, 1995), 13–24.

[37] *Ibid.*, 19.

splitting in terms of a foreclosure of time, of memory, rather than Freud's concept of a splitting of the ego, although Langer does make reference to this as well.

Finally, there is Langer's reference to Nazis and Jews inhabiting different universes of discourse': "…it took the victims a long time to admit this; when they realized it, for most of them it was too late…."[38] Perhaps more disconcertingly, Langer also points out that our 'universe of discourse' is totally different from that of Holocaust survivors. We simply have no comprehension of such a universe; the 'best' we can do is to try to redefine the Holocaust experience in terms of our own discursive universe and give it a "history" and a "narrative".

One of the things that I think stands out when reading Langer's essay is how much his notion of "Holocaust time", what he calls "durational time", chimes with the idea of trauma in general. In other words, perhaps "Holocaust time" is a particular instance of trauma time. After all, is not the whole point about traumatic experiences that they are somehow 'outside' of 'normal', chronological, and historical time? And is not one of the problems for those who have experienced trauma that it just won't go away, that it just keeps repeating itself? In many ways, it doesn't seem quite right to talk of 'traumatic memories', because this sounds like a contradiction in terms; nothing is remembered but rather, it is repeated. If it could be remembered, in the sense of being symbolically processed and transcribed, then it would no longer be traumatic.

The other aspect of trauma I would like to briefly discuss is the idea that *Nachträglichkeit* constitutes the 'mechanism' of history itself. What I mean here is that, as a retroactive process of signification, of 'sense-making', *Nachträglichkeit* constructs the historical narrative at both the individual and at the collective or social level. One example of how this works at the social level is explored in Cathy Caruth's *Unclaimed Experience*, which I referred to briefly in the Introduction, where she uses the term 'belatedness' to describe the idea of retroactive trauma and which is her term for Freud's concept of *Nachträglichkeit*. Caruth's article

[38] *Ibid.*, 20.

is something of a seminal text in the field of trauma studies and, as I noted in the Introduction, has also attracted criticism for being both Eurocentric and for offering an unduly 'pessimistic' account of trauma.[39]

Caruth's central argument is that history fills the 'void' of the Real, of trauma as Real. Not only is history the history *of* trauma, but in a sense, history *as* trauma. She uses the example of Freud's interpretation of the Jewish Exodus in *Moses and Monotheism* to explore this notion.[40] According to Freud, Moses was an aristocratic Egyptian who 'adopted' the captive Hebrew population in Egypt and led them out of their bondage to the promised land of what was then Canaan. Not only that, but he also 'imposed' on them what, according to Freud, was the first monotheistic religion in human history. This was the Atem religion, founded by the Egyptian pharaoh Amenophis III in the Eighteenth Dynasty, and adopted by his son Amenophis IV, who later changed his name to Akhenaten. The Atem religion did not survive the downfall of the Eighteenth Dynasty, but, according to Freud, it found an adherent in Moses. Unfortunately for Moses, having led his 'people' out of captivity, he was then murdered during an uprising, and not only was the deed itself then repressed, but his religion was abandoned. At this point Freud draws upon the work of Eduard Myers who had put forward an alternative history of Moses; one which essentially 'writes out' the Exodus and Moses' early life altogether. In fact, according to Myers, the real Moses was the son-in-law of the Midianite priest Jethro, and who lived in the locality of Meribah-Kadesh in the south of Palestine. The people in this vicinity worshipped the volcano god Yahweh, and Moses of Kadesh was the meditator between Yahweh and the people. According to Freud, the exiles from Egypt encountered the people of Meribah-Kadesh many years later and at this point 'remembered' both the murder of the (Egyptian) Moses and the monotheistic religion he had adopted. This was then 'merged' with the religion of Yahweh and became the foundation of modern Judaism.

---

39 See for example: Visser, 'Decolonizing Trauma Theory', which I also referred to in the Introduction.

40 Sigmund Freud, 'Moses and Monotheism', in *The Standard Edition of the Complete Psychological Works of Sigmund Freud* (London: Hogarth Press, 1939), XXIII, 1–137. XXIII.

Perhaps the most important thing about Freud's 'history' of the Jewish people is not its historical accuracy but rather the way he uses it as an example of a more fundamental theory of trauma, repression and the return of the repressed. And the reason that Cathy Caruth is so interested in Freud's study of Moses is that for her it is a good example of the 'belatedness' of trauma. In his study, Freud uses the idea of *latency* to explain the 'delay' between the initial, traumatic event (the murder of Moses) and the later appearance of pathological symptoms (in this case the development of the Mosaic religion). The term 'latency' equates with Caruth's term 'belatedness' (*Nachträglichkeit*). Freud uses the example of the railway accident which can produce a (delayed) traumatic neurosis. On this point Caruth notes:

> In his use of the term *latency*, the period during which the effects of the experience are not apparent, Freud seems to compare the accident to the successive movement in Jewish history from the event to its repression to its return. Yet what is truly striking about the accident victim's experience of the event, and what in fact constitutes the central enigma revealed by Freud's example, is not so much the period of forgetting that occurs after the accident, but rather the fact that the victim of the crash was never fully conscious during the accident itself: the person gets away, Freud says, "apparently unharmed."[41]

And even more critically, especially in the context of her study of Freud's work:

> The experience of trauma, the fact of latency, would thus seem to consist, not in the forgetting of a reality that can hence never be fully known, but in an inherent latency within the experience itself. The historical power of the trauma is not just that the experience is repeated after its forgetting, *but that it is only in and through its inherent forgetting that it is first experienced at all.*[42]

The event (in this case the murder of Moses) occurs, but is not experienced, is not registered, by the subject(s). The 'registration' can only

[41] Caruth, *Unclaimed Experience*, 17, italics in original.

[42] *Ibid.*, 17, my italics.

occur later on; in the case of Jewish history, according to Freud, at least two generations later (although elsewhere in the text this becomes 'centuries'). But this is not a case of 'delayed' or 'deferred' action. In other words, and this is where perhaps, Freud's use of the term 'repression' is misleading in this context, it is not that later on the Jewish people 'remembered' that they, or rather their ancestors, had murdered Moses. Rather, the story of the murder was constructed *retroactively*. What's more, it *had* to be:

> For history to be a history of trauma means that it is referential precisely to the extent that it is not fully perceived as it occurs; or to put it somewhat differently, that a history can be grasped only in the very inaccessibility of its occurrence.[43]

In other words, history is what fills the 'gap' in lived experience; or rather, lived experience as far as it is registered by the subject. It is important to note here that the history of the Jewish people, as told in the Old Testament, makes no reference to Moses' murder. The most obvious explanation for this is because it never happened and is just pure conjecture on the part of Freud. However, the problem with history, at least in the context of Caruth's argument, is that it can *never* give an account of 'as it really was'. And this is precisely because it is a retroactive process. History is about creating a narrative, a story, of an *absence*, a tear in the fabric of the Symbolic order itself.

[43] *Ibid.*, 18.

7

Conclusion: Psychoanalysis Rehabilitated?

It is now time to pull together, and, in the process, to elaborate upon and clarify, the key arguments that I have discussed in the previous chapters. In doing so my aim is threefold: firstly, to provide the basis for a comprehensive and psychoanalytically based theory of trauma; secondly, to use this theory as a way to challenge the dominant 'mental health' discourse of trauma, which is best exemplified in what I describe as the 'PTSD paradigm'; and thirdly, to briefly address the question as to whether a traumatic neurosis represents a new kind of clinical structure.

Towards a New Understanding of Trauma

In this work I have argued that psychical trauma is the jouissance of the drive (drive-jouissance) that is produced by the continuous circuit of the drive around the object *a*, and which in Lacan's later work is conceptualised as surplus jouissance. Drawing on Miller's idea that surplus jouissance can be seen as the 'crumbs of jouissance' which inhabit the cultural world and through which, according to Miller, "…the body finds the

© The Author(s), under exclusive license to Springer Nature Switzerland AG 2025

L. Chapman, *Traumatic Neurosis Revisited*, The Palgrave Lacan Series,
https://doi.org/10.1007/978-3-031-89158-8_7

wherewithal to feed its jouissance and lack of jouissance",[1] my argument is that such a 'feeding' is the basis of psychical trauma.

The signifier produces traces on the body which produces jouissance which in turn produces trauma because the pleasure principle is unable to regulate the excitation produced by such jouissance. This is not only Miller's argument but is also the core thesis of my work. However, this is only part of the story. The incessant tracing of the body by the signifier continues for the life of the human being[2] and this is effected through the continuous repetition of the drive. But as I noted in Chap. 3, the repetition of the drive is the repetition of the signifier itself, which is continuously both creating and destroying the network of signification that constitutes the Symbolic register. And if we refer back to the idea that I explored in Chap. 4 regarding the relation between *automaton* and *tuché*, the *automaton* seems to be in a somewhat paradoxical position because of the one hand it provides the framework for the Symbolic register through the construction of binary codes (what Liu describes as the 'cybernetic unconscious') which operate in a cybernetic and repetitive fashion; and yet on the other hand there is another 'repetition' operating here that undermines that of the *automaton*, and this is work of the *tuché*.

As I noted in Chap. 4 it is by no means clear why Lacan argues that the *automaton* is not repetition whereas the *tuché* is, but perhaps one way to think about this is to use the concept of *entropy* that I touched upon in Chaps. 2 and 4. It will be recalled that in cybernetics the idea of *negative* entropy is used to explain how any system of circulating symbols tends towards organisation and order, rather than the disorder and randomness which is the characteristic of *positive* entropy (or simply 'entropy'). This would suggest that it is not repetition per se that is characteristic of the *tuché*, but rather something that disrupts the stabilising and organisational function of repetition; and it should be remembered that what are being stabilised and organised through repetition are *signifiers*.

---

[1] Miller, *Six Paradigms*, 61.

[2] And beyond to the extent the dead body becomes immortalised through its entombment. As Alexandre Stevens notes: "The dead body is not simply carrion, the signifier has elevated it to a singular dimension that deserves to be captured in a funerary organization. Burial signifies a permanence of the body beyond life." Alexandre Stevens, "The Bodily Effects of Language", 2. Paper delivered at the NLS Congress, May 2020.

And yet, as I discussed in Chap. 5, the repetition of the signifier is what produces jouissance; a jouissance that is perpetually 'running down' so that all that remains is the object *a*, surplus jouissance. So it would seem that the repetition of the signifier produces both (positive) entropy and negative entropy at the same time; and this appears to be in line with Lacan's argument at the end of *Seminar II* regarding the death drive as the Symbolic order in the process of becoming. And it is important to note that although Lacan referred in *Seminar XVII* to jouissance as 'running down', being subject to entropy, strictly speaking it does not actually *disappear*. It is still present in the living body, but is not (always) accessible to the subject, who has to make do with Miller's 'crumbs of jouissance', that is, surplus jouissance.

But where *is* the subject in all this? So far in this section my focus has been on the (lost) jouissance of the body and its relation to trauma rather than the subject of jouissance (and trauma). However, the subject is not the same as the body—or is it? The only reason I raise this question is that by the time we get to the 'late' Lacan the status of human subject appears to become increasingly problematic. Or, rather, the exact relationship between the subject and the body becomes increasingly problematic. As Miller reminds us, the 'classical' reading of Lacan (although he does not use this term) is that the subject *has* a body rather than *being* a body: "If we can identify being and body for the animal, we cannot do the same for the human species. As far as the speaking body is concerned, it does not emerge from being but from having."[3] But even here there appears to be a contradiction: Miller does not refer to the speaking *subject*, but rather the speaking *body*. So is he arguing that the speaking body emerges from having … a body? At this point it is important to note that Miller (in *Lacanian Biology*) makes reference to Cartesian dualism:

> The dualism here is of knowledge and of body. The question of being for "man" is posed on the side of knowledge, while the body is on the side of having. This identification of man with his knowledge is what made Lacan

[3] Miller, *Lacanian Biology*, 15.

> culminate with the concept of the algorithm of the subject. His position is on the order of being, even if it is formulated as lack-in-being.[4]

Miller goes on to note that the subject "…from the moment in which it is subject of the signifier, cannot identify itself as its body, and it is precisely from there that its affection for the image of its body proceeds."[5] It seems clear from this passage that the 'body' in question is the *Imaginary* body rather than the *speaking* one, which is also the body of jouissance.

But as far as *trauma* is concerned, which subject (and which body) is at stake? Referring back to my discussion in Chap. 4, it will be recalled that Lacan's argument in *Science and Truth* was that the subject of psychoanalysis is the subject of modern science. And if, as Lacan indicates in *Seminar XI*, the *automaton* is the network of signifiers, we can perhaps refer to the *automaton* of modern science; in other words, the discourse of modern science. Furthermore, it would seem that the discourse of modern science, based on mathematics, is the *automaton par excellence*. In other words, the idea of the *automaton* as the endless circuit of signifiers encoded in binary numbers which can be formulated in the language of cybernetics and computer science.

The moment of modern science, according to Lacan, is the moment of the Cartesian subject (which, as I argued in Chap. 4, pre-dates the historical Descartes). A Cartesian subject that, argues Lacan, is less 'Cartesian' than it first appears. A subject that, according to Miller's argument in his *Suture* paper, 'vanishes' under the signifier to be replaced by the 'stand-in' subject of the signifying chain. However, the subject has not really 'vanished' at all; rather, it reappears as the subject of the Real, the subject of trauma, the subject of jouissance. And it is this subject of the Real, this subject of jouissance, that is the subject of psychoanalysis. Furthermore, insofar that life, the living body, is the condition of jouissance (Miller's argument) then the subject of psychoanalysis is the body itself; not, of course, the Imaginary body, the body of the Mirror Stage, but, rather, the body of jouissance.

---

[4] *Ibid.*, 15–16.

[5] *Ibid.*, 16.

This body is also, according to Miller's argument in *Six Paradigms of Jouissance*, jouissance One, jouissance without the Other. As Miller points out:

> One can even hear the title of *Encore* [*Seminar XX*] as a homophone, as Lacan suggests at one point—*En-corps*. It is the body that is at stake here, far more than the repetition he spoke of his *The Other Side of Psychoanalysis* [*Seminar XVII*] in the marriage of jouissance and knowledge.[6]

At this point it is worth noting that this subject, jouissance One, is very different from the subject of language, insofar that by 'language' we mean the signifying network. This latter subject is in a relation to the Other, the Other of language, the Other of the unconscious. In this sense the Other is a necessary condition of this subject; but not of the subject of jouissance. And if we go back to the idea of the *automaton* of modern science then perhaps it is not so obvious after all that the existence (or even better, the ek-sistence) of the Other is as certain as we think it is. In other words, in a world of mathematical equations and logical propositions, that is, the discourse of modern science, it is by no means clear where (or what) the Other is. All that seems certain, in a rather paradoxical manner, is the *in-sistence* of subject of the Real, of jouissance One. In the 'classical Lacan' the Other essentially 'resided' in the structure of language, in the Symbolic register. But, as Miller points out: "'Structure is full of holes and, in these holes, there is room for invention, for novelty, for connections that have not always been there'. However, he goes onto argue: 'This does not mean that there is no structure, that everything is semblance. There is the real, but it is much more difficult today than formerly to isolate and discern what is structure and what is real.'"[7] In other words, the ek-sistence of the Other, at least in terms of the Symbolic register, of structure, becomes highly problematic.

There is, however, still the question of the *drive* and its relation to jouissance. In Chap. 5 I argued that the drive is essentially the 'motor force' of both the signifier and of jouissance. In Freud's work, and especially

[6] Miller, *Six Paradigms*, 70–71.

[7] *Ibid.*, 77.

Inhibitions, Symptoms and Anxiety, one gets the impression that the drive is something 'internal' to the subject; or, more precisely, perhaps, to the human organism. At the same time, though, Freud described the drive as a 'frontier concept' between the psychical and the somatic, and Lacan went even further to describe it as a 'montage'. There is also the fact that Freud, somewhat implicitly in *Beyond the Pleasure Principle* and more explicitly in *Inhibitions, Symptoms and Anxiety*, argued that trauma, as excess excitation, emanated from both 'external' and 'internal' sources. But in the context of trauma, what exactly is 'external' and what is 'internal'? Or, to put it another way, where is the *source* of the surplus-jouissance that is traumatising the subject?

As I noted earlier, in his *Six Paradigms* essay Miller refers to the 'crumbs of jouissance' that inhabit the cultural world. Such 'crumbs' are all that remains of the 'lost' jouissance of the body; both a *remainder* and a *reminder* of a lost rapture. And my contention is that in its relentless quest to regain such 'lost' jouissance the drive is perpetually 'scraping'[8] the cultural world for yet more 'crumbs'. Furthermore, I would argue, in a cultural world that is becoming increasingly saturated by such 'crumbs of jouissance', for example through social media and a 24/7 news cycle, the subject finds it increasingly difficult to decipher the perpetual overload of enjoyment (surplus jouissance). And what remains ciphered, what escapes meaning, is trauma. However, a key part of this argument hinges around the idea that the drive and culture are not as diametrically opposed as they may appear to be. This is in spite of the fact that, as Mladen Dolar points out in his paper on this topic, it is all too easy to read Freud this way, for example in *Civilisation and its Discontents*.[9] Dolar argues that culture and the drive are intertwined in six different ways (which he describes as the 'six fundamental traits of the drive'), and these are (1) as the mastery of nature, (2) as the non-functional supplement (the inverse of (1)); (3) the drive towards cleanliness, which Dolar links to the anal

[8] I am using the term 'scraping' here as an analogy of 'web scraping', which is the process whereby computer programs extract or 'scrape' information from web sites. For a (reasonably) academic introduction to this process see: Nicholas J DeVito, Georgia C Richards, and Peter Inglesby, 'How We Learnt to Stop Worrying and Love Web Scraping', *Nature*, 585.7826 (2020), 621–22.

[9] Mladen Dolar, 'Of Drives and Culture', in *Analyzing the Cultural Unconscious: Science of the Signifier*, ed. by Henrik Bjerre and others (London: Bloomsbury Academic, 2020), 69–86.

drive); (4) the drive towards order, which Dolar links to the compulsion to repeat; (5) spiritual elevation, which he links to sublimation; (6) the renunciation of satisfaction, which as Dolar notes, following Lacan, is precisely the drive's *means* of satisfaction. In terms of my own argument, there a number of overlaps with Dolar's. For example, the drive's continuous repetition, which, paradoxically becomes its mode of satisfaction; and the idea of the 'supplementary' nature of the drive's object. Dolar's argument here is that one way to view culture is precisely in terms of its *non-utility*, its 'uselessness': "The moment of expenditure, of the non-functional, of waste, which defies the logic of self-preservation and survival, is the true breeding ground of culture."[10] There seem to be strong echoes here of the idea of a surplus (supplementary) enjoyment (jouissance), which appears to undermine a strictly utilitarian concept of culture, that is, one that functions to ensure human survival. With regards to this apparent dichotomy between the utilitarian and the 'non-functional Dolar comments:

> The two first traits form a paradoxical couple: on the one hand, culture as the maximization of utility, and on the other hand, culture as uselessness, pure expenditure. Is culture something that serves best or something that doesn't serve at all? Utility or futility? The maximum purpose or no purpose at all? But purpose for what, in view of what?[11]

In many ways this seems to be another way of describing the (apparent) dichotomy between the pleasure principle and its 'beyond' (the Other jouissance). This is also, perhaps, a way to read Freud's *Civilisation and its Discontents*.[12] Freud's basic argument here was the price of civilisation (and it is important to note that the German title of the work is *Das Unbehagen in der Kultur*) is the renunciation of the (direct) satisfaction of the drives. In other words, ensuring that the pleasure principle fulfils its function. But as Lacan realised, the idea of a 'direct' satisfaction of the

[10] *Ibid.* 74.

[11] *Ibid.* 75.

[12] Sigmund Freud, "Civilisation and Its Discontents," in *The Standard Edition of the Complete Psychological Works of Sigmund Freud*, vol. XXI (London: Hogarth Press, 1930), 59–145.

drive(s) was something of a misnomer; rather, the drive's 'satisfaction' lay precisely in its eternal repetition, its 'non-satisfaction'. In this reading, 'civilisation' (*Kultur*) becomes the site for the enactment of the (death) drive rather than the renunciation of it.

There is, however, one other aspect of trauma that we need to incorporate into a psychoanalytic theory of trauma, and this is the question of *Nachträglichkeit*. In Chap. 6 I argued that Freud developed this idea in order to explain the rather curious fact that certain events that occurred in a subject's early history were not at the time of their occurrence registered as 'traumatic'. Rather, it was only at a later date (which Freud argued was post-puberty) and in the wake of another event that was associated with the 'original' one that the subject became traumatised. I went on to argue that this is not, in spite of Strachey's translation of *Nachträglichkeit* as 'deferred action', a matter of a 'delayed' trauma or an 'original' trauma that was 'triggered' by the occurrence of the later event. Rather, the trauma is constructed *retroactively*; in other words, the trauma is an effect of the chain of association that is constructed in the present, which means there is no 'original' trauma. I then discussed Laplanche's approach to *Nachträglichkeit* and how he used it as part of his broader theory of childhood seduction. He argued that the young child is 'seduced' by another person (often but not always an adult) and that part of this 'seduction' takes the form of enigmatic messages regarding the other's jouissance being conveyed to the child. The 'seduced' subject then spends many years, if not a lifetime, trying to make sense of these enigmatic messages through a series of failed translations retroactively constructed. It is the failure of each translation that perpetuates the trauma for the subject.

The key point to remember here is that *Nachträglichkeit* is a purely retroactive phenomenon and that this contradicts Laplanche's assertion that *Nachträglichkeit* is 'bidirectional'. His argument was that the enigmatic messages that the other conveys to the infant subject take place in chronological ('forward moving) time whereas the subject's (failed) attempts at translation take place retroactively. However, my argument is that Laplanche's idea theory of childhood seduction is itself a retroactive construction in order to explain the subsequent series of failed translations. This is not to argue for one moment that something never happened to the subject; something that in many cases would probably nowadays be considered child abuse. However, the whole point about *Nachträglichkeit* is that it becomes impossible to say what 'really' happened. Clearly, the same argument could be applied to Freud's original theory of childhood seduction, although interestingly enough it was not one of the reasons he gave in his letter to Fliess for 'abandoning' this theory.

In my view, the critical point about *Nachträglichkeit* is that it is a way to theorise the failure of the narration of the trauma. Whether we use Freud's concept of re-transcription or Laplanche's concept of re-translation, what is at stake here is the idea that something fails in the subject's attempt to make sense of an experience in their history. In fact, the attempt at sense-making is an attempt to *construct* a history in the first place. In this sense, *all* history is a process of *Nachträglichkeit*, whether on an individual or collective scale, which is why I discussed the example of Caruth's reading of Freud's *Moses and Monotheism* in the previous chapter. But at some point, all these narratives, all these histories, fail; something always escapes meaning, and that something is surplus jouissance, which is the source of the trauma.

But *why*? Why does something always escape symbolisation, escape meaning? In my view there are two possible explanations. The first is what might be called the 'deficit model' of narrativisation. The process of giving meaning, of creating narratives, is simply unable to cope with the excess jouissance that is continually impacting on the subject. This is one way to interpret Freud's argument in *Beyond the Pleasure Principle*: trauma is the result of the 'protective shield' of the psychical apparatus becoming overwhelmed by excitations from the outside world and in the process the pleasure principle is put out action. In Lacanian terms this means that the regulatory function of language breaks down. On this reading the traumatic neuroses are the effect of an overload of excitation (Lacan's jouissance) on the subject. The implication here is that a bit more narrativisation, a bit more therapy, a bit more storytelling, will finally 'capture' the Real of the trauma and turn it into a coherent trauma narrative. The problem with this approach is that experience would suggest otherwise. No matter how much trauma is narrativised, no matter how much therapy is undertaken, no matter how many stories are told, the trauma persists. In fact, if anything it seems to become ever more pervasive; as I argued above, the cultural world seems to be more and more saturated with surplus jouissance, more and more inhabited with sites of trauma.

One way to explain this apparent paradox, that is, that more narrativisation produces more trauma, is to remember what Lacan said in *Seminar XVII* about knowledge as a means of jouissance. As I discussed in Chap. 5 this is linked to the idea that the signifier is an apparatus of jouissance. This seems to suggest that jouissance is 'wired-in' to knowledge, and therefore into narrativisation. In other words, the more stories that are told, the more history (hystory) that is produced, the greater the amount of jouissance. (Trauma) narratives fail not because of some 'deficit' in the narrative, some inability to 'capture' the Real of the trauma, but, rather, because jouissance, that is trauma, is 'built into' the narrative itself. Perhaps this should not come as such a surprise if we go back to Miller's argument in *Lacanian Biology* regarding the living body as the condition of jouissance. It is not only the living body that is the condition of jouissance, it is the *speaking* body as well. This idea is reinforced by Miller's remarks in his *Body Event* paper in relation to the Schreber case:

> But it is in the Schreber case that one can find the paradigm that thought is *jouissance*. This proposition, which Lacan will formulate a long afterwards, is delivered there clearly, including the concept that speech is *jouissance*, since Schreber's incessant thought is especially manifested by an articulated cogitation, eventually expressed.[13]

In other words, not only was Schreber's discourse *concerning* jouissance (and especially the jouissance of God), but it was also *laden* with jouissance, it was an *apparatus* of jouissance. And this is also the case, I would argue, with much therapeutic discourse, for example, in the (trauma) narratives that are recounted every day in consulting rooms around the globe. Although it is certainly the case that such narratives can have a calming effect on the subject, they are also *carriers* of jouissance, albeit often repressed. And it is clearly the case that other forms of representation, including the written word, film, music, and so on, are also apparatus of jouissance. This is perhaps especially true nowadays with the

[13] Miller, *The Symptom and the Body Event*, 33.

explosion of 'speech-like' discourses, for example, WhatsApp and X (formerly Twitter) messages, Facebook and Instagram posts, and so on. However, there still appears to be a widespread view within the psychoanalytic world that privileges the spoken word and this is something Shirley Zisser explores in some depth in her book on writing, speech and the body.[14] It could also be the case that such a privileging of the spoken word is part of the legacy of the 'Saussurian Lacan' that I discussed in Chap. 3. This is somewhat ironic, bearing in mind that, as Zisser is keen to point out, not only did Freud not privilege speech in this way but in his later work Lacan himself became much more interested in the written word, for example in *Seminar XVIII*[15] and *Seminar XX*. On the other hand, and as Derrida was keen to point out, for example in his text *Plato's Pharmacy*, the privileging of speech over writing goes back a lot further than Saussure.[16] Therefore, it may be some time before a broader understanding of the 'jouissance of the narrative' is fully established.

Why Traumatic Neurosis, Whither PTSD?

But where does traumatic neurosis fit into all this? And what about PTSD, which still appears to be the dominant 'trauma paradigm' of the early part of the twenty-first century? With regards to the first question, I am essentially following (and, in the process, re-reading) Freud, and especially his arguments in *Beyond the Pleasure Principle* and in *Inhibitions, Symptoms and Anxiety*. This is his idea that a traumatic neurosis is the result of excess excitation which overwhelms the regulatory function of the pleasure principle. In Lacanian terms this can be conceptualised as the irruption of the Real, in the form of drive-jouissance, into the Symbolic-Imaginary construction that forms the subject's 'reality' and which also constitutes 'culture'. A key part of this argument hinges on the

[14] Shirley Zisser, *Writing, Speech and Flesh in Lacanian Psychoanalysis: Of Unconscious Grammatology* (Abingdon, Oxon: Routledge, 2022).

[15] Jacques Lacan, *The Seminar of Jacques Lacan Book XVIII 1971: On a Discourse That Might Not Be a Semblance*, trans. Cormac Gallagher (Dublin: Unpublished translation by Cormac Gallagher, 2011).

[16] Jacques Derrida, "Plato's Pharmacy," in *Dissemination* (London: The Athlone Press, 1981).

idea of there being no clear demarcation between drive and culture, or between the 'internal' and 'external'. It is my contention that the traumatic neuroses demonstrate that there is a direct relationship between the trauma of the drive, which continues for the life of the subject, and so-called 'external traumas', which I have chosen to call the 'wounds of life'.

The critical point here is that t*he human subject is always already traumatised by the operation of the drive, but in 'normal' circumstances such a trauma is mitigated by the regulatory function of the pleasure principle.* However, there are circumstances, which, I would argue, are becoming increasingly 'normalised', where the trauma of the drive, that is, drive-jouissance, overwhelms the operation of the pleasure principle. At this point a traumatic neurosis will appear. The reason I argue that the circumstances that lead to an overwhelming of the pleasure principle are becoming increasingly 'normalised' links back to my earlier argument that the cultural world is becoming saturated with sites of surplus-jouissance, that is, trauma. Consequently, traumatic neurosis itself is becoming 'normalised'. Does this mean, though, that the traumatic neuroses should now be included as a clinical structure within the Lacanian clinic, alongside those of neurosis, perversion[17] and psychosis? The short answer is no, but before elaborating I would now like to address the second question that I posed at the start of this section regarding the currently dominant position of the 'PTSD paradigm'.

To begin with I think it is important to reflect a bit more upon why such a paradigm is currently very much the dominant one, at least in Western mental health discourse. As I pointed out in the Introduction, PTSD is essentially a product of the politics of the aftermath of the Vietnam War, and, perhaps to a slightly lesser extent, the politics of Holocaust survival.[18] According to this argument, trauma is something that can happen to anyone, and, primarily, is the result of external events that impose themselves on individuals, groups, or even whole societies. In other words, we are all victims or potential victims of trauma, as opposed to being perpetrators of acts of violence that inflict psychological

[17] In some Lacanian schools, especially those of a Millerian orientation, perversion has effectively disappeared as a clinical structure for reasons that are not totally clear.

[18] And also the influence of *feminism* (see chp 4 of Fassin and Rechtman's *The Empire of Trauma*).

and physical injury on others, and which (may) produce feelings of guilt and remorse And even if we substitute my preferred term, that is, 'wounds of life' for the more commonly used 'traumatic events', in practical terms this does not appear to change the thrust of the argument. It is also important to stress that at the level of symptomatology there appears to be little to distinguish traumatic neurosis from PTSD, and much of the contemporary literature on trauma appears to treat the two as synonymous, for example Fassin and Rechtman whom I referenced in the Introduction. They note that the "…semiological outlines of PTSD were virtually identical to classic descriptions of traumatic neurosis, merely refining and stabilizing the criteria for the diagnosis."[19]

But if this is the case, why bother inventing a new diagnostic category (PTSD) when there is already a near identical one (the traumatic neuroses)? Is it purely down to politics (and ideology), whereby psychoanalysis is simply no longer deemed relevant in the clinic of trauma, or at least not in its more radical Freudian and Lacanian guises? In my view, the answer is most likely 'yes'; that is, the dominance of the PTSD paradigm over the psychoanalytic has a great deal to do with politics and ideology, but such a dominance is sustained by a fundamental misunderstanding of the relationship between the traumatic neuroses and PTSD. If Fassin and Rechtman are right in their argument that the semiological outlines (symptomatology) of traumatic neurosis and PTSD are pretty much identical then it would appear that the only grounds for choosing one over the other would be down to personal preference or, more likely, the prevalence of a particular discourse of trauma, and, in a broader sense, of 'mental health' in general. However, I argue that there is more at stake here than simply the question of terminology (or, indeed, politics). Although superficially the traumatic neuroses and PTSD may look the same, there is a crucial difference.

Referring back to the brief quote above from Fassin and Rechtman, they immediately go onto to argue that:

> The first (diagnostic) criterion (of PTSD), however, was a major departure. It effectively affirmed that any normal individual might suffer from such

[19] Fassin and Rechtman, *The Empire of Trauma*, 77.

> distress if he or she were exposed to an event deemed traumatic. This marked a complete reversal in attitude. There was no longer any need to posit a weak personality, since the symptoms represented a statistically normal reaction to the event. There was no need to seek out any original trauma, since the event alone was sufficient to produce the distress.[20]

Furthermore, such distressed (traumatised) individuals are *victims*. As I noted in the Introduction, and particularly in relation to El-Haj's arguments, *everyone* is now a victim or potential victim, even those whose role it is to inflict violence upon others, for example, soldiers, terrorists, and other perpetrators. And, furthermore, trauma victims 'require' events that are 'external' to them, otherwise the very nature of their 'victimhood' is called into question. In other words, victims must not in any way be 'culpable' or bear some responsibility for their victimhood. And it is this correlation between 'victimhood' and the 'externality' of trauma that I believe is critical in understanding the true difference between my reconfiguration of the traumatic neuroses in this work and PTSD. But to be clear, I am not for one moment suggesting that subjects of trauma are in some way 'to blame' for their situation. To do so would be to miss the essential point of my argument, which is that human subjects are *always already traumatised*. What I have aimed to do in this work is to explore how exactly such a traumatisation comes about, and, more crucially, how it is *sustained* through the incessant operation of the drive.

And this brings me back to the question of whether the traumatic neuroses represent a clinical structure. At this point it might be helpful to refer back to Gault's paper that I cited earlier, where he argues that in cases of neurosis there is a movement in the analysis from the Symbolic to the Real in order, as Miller puts it, to bring "…the subject back to his truly elementary signifiers, on which he has, in his neurosis, had a delusion."[21] This implies, of course, that for the neurotic subject, the delusion is already in place; a delusion that is enabled by the 'anchoring' of the master signifier of the Name-of-the-Father. And another name for this delusion is the *sinthome*, which Lacan explores in great depth in

[20] *Ibid.*, 77.

[21] Jacques-Alain Miller, 'Interpretation in Reverse', in *The Later Lacan: An Introduction*, ed. by Véronique Voruz and Bogdan Wolf (State of New York: Sunny Press, 2007), 7.

Seminar XXIII.[22] Put somewhat simplistically, the sinthome is a 'knotting together' of the Real, Symbolic and Imaginary. For the neurotic subject, such a knotting together is established through the subject's entry into language. In fact, in his *Joyce the Symptom* lecture in 1975 Lacan argued that the Name-of-the-Father is a sinthome, so essentially the neurosis itself functions as a sinthome.[23]

In the case of psychosis, the delusion, the sinthome, has to be constructed in the here-and-now, and this is effected, argues Gault, by a movement from the Real to the Symbolic. As Jean-Claude Maleval explains:

> It is important to take seriously Freud's discovery that the delusion is already an attempt at a cure. The delusion constitutes a metaphor that functions as a *suppléance* to the foreclosed paternal metaphor so that in its most elaborate forms (paranoid and paraphrenic) it succeeds in framing the subject's jouissance. Wedded to idealized signifiers, it can stabilize reality. At times it happens that a favorable end of a psychotic cure can in fact be the structuration of a delusion.[24]

The term *suppléance* is an important concept which, as I noted above, in *Seminar XXIII* Lacan develops in terms of the *sinthome* and argues that Joyce's writing functioned as a way to 'knot' together the Real, Symbolic and Imaginary. More generally it is related to the idea in Lacanian psychoanalysis that it is possible to 'stabilise' the psychotic subject through the construction of what could perhaps be described as a 'prosthetic Symbolic', that is, a construction of meaning that regulates jouissance. But isn't this essentially the same as the construction of a trauma narrative in the form of a delusion? And doesn't it also raise the question as to whether what I have been describing as traumatic neurosis is, in fact, psychosis? In other words, if traumatic neurosis can be thought of in

---

[22] Jacques Lacan, *The Sinthome: The Seminar of Jacques Lacan, Book XXIII*, ed. Jacques-Alain Miller (Cambridge: Polity Press, 2016).

[23] Jacques Lacan, "Joyce the Symptom," in *The Seminar of Jacques Lacan Book XXIII 1975–76: The Sinthome*, ed. Jacques-Alain Miller (Cambridge: Polity Press, 2016), 141–48.

[24] Jean-Claude Maleval, "Treatment of the Psychosis and Contemporary Psychoanalysis," in *Lacan on Madness: Madness, Yes You Can't*, ed. Patricia Gherovici and Steinkoler (Hove: Routledge, 2015), 106.

terms of an irruption of the Real into the Symbolic-Imaginary, isn't this precisely what happens in psychosis? From this perspective, traumatic neurosis is not a clinical structure but, rather, the description of a psychotic break.

However, just to complicate things even more, within Lacanian psychoanalysis, and especially within Millerian circles, there is an increasing questioning of some of the basic tenets of the 'differential clinic' itself, that is, the distinction between neurosis and psychosis.[25] This is particularly the case where the focus is on the teachings of the 'very late Lacan', that is, of the late 1970s and Lacan's proposition that "everyone is mad, that is, delusional."[26] The trajectory of the (Millerian) argument here seems to be that neurosis itself is a form of delusion and functions as a *suppléance* or sinthome. For example, François Sauvagnat argues that the child Hans in Freud's Little Hans case study employed the signifier of the horse as a *suppléance* for the debased father function, even though Hans has always been regarded as a *neurotic* subject.[27] That being said, not all contemporary Lacanians subscribe to this reading of Lacan. David Ferraro, for example, is quite scathing in his critique of the 'wilder' interpretations of Miller's work. For example, he argues that the statement 'everyone is mad':

> …if it is not merely a rhetorical provocation, stands as a repudiation of structure and paradigmatic shifts. If the delusion in question is identification with the ego, with all the narcissism implied by this, then this slogan merely recapitulates Lacan's Schema L from the 1950s in which the ego is clearly distinct from the subject. It is equivalent to asserting that there is an imaginary register, which is to say that it stays at the level of the insights of 70 years ago.[28]

---

[25] Although to be fair to Miller, this does not appear to be a position he himself subscribes to.

[26] Jacques Lacan, "There Are Four Discourses," *Culture/Clinic*, no. 1 (2013): 3–4. For an interesting discussion of these ideas see Pierre-Gilles Guéguen, 'Who Is Mad and Who Is Not? On Differential Diagnosis in Psychoanalysis', *Culture/Clinic*, 1 (2013), 66–85.

[27] François Sauvagnat, "Fatherhood and Naming in J. Lacan's Works," The Symptom, 3, 2002, https://www.lacan.com/fathernamef.htm

[28] David Ferraro, "Some Further Questions Prior to Any Possible Treatment of the Psychoses," *Psychoanalysis Lacan* 6 (2023): 69–76.

This reflects Ferraro's deeper scepticism regarding attempts, especially amongst the Millerian school, to 'prioritise' the (very) late teachings of Lacan at the expense of his earlier, more structuralist based work; and in doing so to effectively abandon the idea of a differential clinic and, along with it, the key role played by the signifier of the Name-of-the-Father in determining clinical structure.

But going back to my original question, in what way is a traumatic neurosis different from a psychosis? As Maleval reminds us, from 1967 onwards Lacan increasingly emphasised the role that a 'deregulated' jouissance played in destabilising the subject and on the face of it this would seem to apply equally to traumatic neurosis. This seems tantamount to arguing that a traumatic neurosis is either, as I hinted at earlier, a psychotic break in someone with a psychotic structure, or some form of 'temporary psychosis'. But perhaps it could be equally be argued that a psychosis is a form of 'permanent' or 'prolonged' traumatic neurosis, but in a sense this is something of a red herring. The key point is the degree to which jouissance is regulated, deciphered; and on the whole the neurotic subject seems to fare better in this respect than the psychotic. But if we are to take the (Millerian) readings of the 'late Lacan' seriously, and not withstanding Ferraro's objections, then all this is saying is that neurosis (perhaps) provides a more robust form of the sinthome than does the delusion. Traumatic neurosis, on the other hand, is essentially on the other side of the equation, so to speak; it represents the irruption of jouissance into the subject which the neurosis and the delusion both try to counter. In other words, traumatic neurosis has nothing to do with clinical structure per se, but, rather, is a way of describing the mechanism by which the pleasure principle breaks down.

What, though, of the 'wounds of life' that I argue have the capacity to overwhelm the regulatory function of the pleasure principle? Are they not 'traumatic' in their own right? Take, for example, the question of the war neuroses, which were the precursor to PTSD and the focus of much of Freud's later work on the traumatic neuroses. Is not being constantly shelled and bombed, crouching helplessly for days or weeks on end in filthy trenches and dugouts, being surrounded by death and serious injury, and even being subjected to one's own (physical) wounding, traumatic in itself? The short answer is yes—*but only to the extent that such 'wounds' impact on the operation of the pleasure principle*; or, to put it in more Lacanian terms, only to the extent that such 'wounds' disrupt the functioning of language in regulating jouissance. But to be clear, such 'wounds' are rooted in the signifier; the signifier that is continually 'tracing' (to use Miller's term) the flesh of the body. And this applies to *any* 'life wounding event'. The central point of my entire argument is that such wounds all form part of the 'inaugural' trauma that constitutes the human subject. Just to reiterate: such an 'inauguration' is not a 'one-off' occurrence but a continuous process effected by the operation of the drive. In other words, there is no separate trauma that gives birth to the subject; rather, it is the incessant repetition of the drive as it continually 'scrapes' the world for surplus jouissance that perpetually traumatises the subject. For much of the time, such a perpetual traumatisation is kept in check by the homeostatic function of the pleasure principle, but on occasion such a function breaks down and then the jouissance of the drive is given free rein. And one of the tragic ironies of attempts to 'cure' trauma through giving meaning to meaningless ('traumatic') experiences, often through the construction of various forms of trauma narrative, is that such meanings, such narratives, contain within themselves the seeds of their own destruction. This is because of the nature of language itself, which is ultimately rooted in the jouissance of the signifier, and which means that constructions of language, including trauma narratives, beget more jouissance, more trauma.

This is not to deny that such trauma narratives have no therapeutic or calming effects; clearly they do. However, the idea that trauma can be 'narrativised' away, either at the individual level through, for example, psychotherapy, or at the more collective level through historical narratives, is an illusion. And perhaps one of the key roles that psychoanalysis can fulfil within the field of trauma is to show *why* it is an illusion; and, leading on from this, to redefine the place of trauma within the human condition.

Bibliography

Ahbel-Rappe, Karin. "'I No Longer Believe': Did Freud Abandon the Seduction Theory?" *Journal of the American Psychoanalytic Association* 54, no. 1 (March 1, 2006): 171–99.

Aho, Kevin. "Ek-Sistence (Ek-Sisntenz)." In *The Cambridge Heidegger Lexicon*, edited by Mark Wrathall, 268–70. Cambridge: Cambridge University Press, 2021.

Alexander, Jeffrey C. *Trauma: A Social Theory*. Cambridge: Polity Press, 2012.

Allen, James. "Aristotle on Chance as an Accidental Cause." In *Aristotle's Physics: A Critical Guide*, edited by Mariska Leunissen, 66–87. Cambridge Critical Guides. Cambridge: Cambridge University Press, 2015.

Angermuller, Johannes. *Why There Is No Poststructuralism in France The Making of an Intellectual Generation*. London: Bloomsbury Academic, 2015.

Aristotle. *Physics*. Oxford: Oxford University Press, 1996.

Bistoen, Gregory, Stijn Vanheule, and Stef Craps. "Nachträglichkeit: A Freudian Perspective on Delayed Traumatic Reactions." *Theory and Psychology*, 2014, 1–20.

Boothby, Richard. *Death and Desire: Psychoanalytic Theory in Lacan's Return to Freud*. Hove: Routledge, 1991.

Braunstein, Néstor A. *Jouissance A Lacanian Concept*. New York: Suny Press, 2020.

© The Author(s), under exclusive license to Springer Nature Switzerland AG 2025

L. Chapman, *Traumatic Neurosis Revisited*, The Palgrave Lacan Series,
https://doi.org/10.1007/978-3-031-89158-8

Budryte, Dovile. "Decolonization of Trauma and Memory Politics: Insights from Eastern Europe." In *Decolonizing Trauma Studies: Trauma and Postcolonialism*, edited by Sonya Andermahr, 153–68. Switzerland: MDPI—Multidisciplinary Digital Publishing Institute, 2016.

Cantin, Lucie. "The Trauma of Language." In *After Lacan: Clinical Practice and the Subject of the Unconscious*, edited by Robert Hughes and Kareen Malone, 35–47. Albany: State University of New York Press, 2002.

Caruth, Cathy. *Unclaimed Experience: Trauma, Narrative and History*. John Hopkins University Press, 1996.

Charlton, William. *Aristotle Physics Books I and II*. Oxford: Clarendon Press, 1970.

Collins, Dan. "Debunking the Drive." In *Critical Essays on the Drive: Lacanian Theory and Practice*, edited by Dan Collins and Eve Watson, 1–39. The Lines of the Symbolic in Psychoanalysis Series. Abingdon, Oxon: Routledge, 2024.

Derrida, Jacques. *Of Grammatology*. Corrected Edition. Baltimore: The Johns Hopkins University Press, 1997.

———. "Plato's Pharmacy." In *Dissemination*. London: The Athlone Press, 1981.

Descartes, René. *A Discourse on Method/ Meditations on the First Philosophy/ Principles of Philosophy*. London: Everyman's Library, 1912.

DeVito, Nicholas J., Georgia C. Richards, and Peter Inglesby. "How We Learnt to Stop Worrying and Love Web Scraping." *Nature* 585, no. 7826 (September 2020): 621–22.

Dolar, Mladen. "Of Drives and Culture." In *Analyzing the Cultural Unconscious: Science of the Signifier (Kindle Edition)*, edited by Henrik Bjerre, Brian Hansen, Kirsten Hyldgaard, Jakob Rosendale, and Lilian Rösing, 69–86. London: Bloomsbury Academic, 2020.

Dor, Joël. *Introduction to the Reading of Lacan: The Unconscious Is Structured Like a Language*. New York: The Other Press, 1998.

Dravers, Philip. "The Drive as a Fundamental Concept of Psychoanalysis." *Psychoanalytical Notebooks*, no. 23 (September 2011): 117–49.

El-Haj, Nadia Abu. *Combat Trauma: Imaginaries of War and Citizenship in Post-9/11 America (Kindle Edition)*. London: Verso, 2002.

Ellenberger, Henri. "Fechner and Freud." *Bulletin of the Menninger Clinic* 20, no. 4 (1956): 201–14.

Evans, Dylan. *An Introductory Dictionary of Lacanian Psychoanalysis*. London: Routledge, 1996.

Faimberg, Haydée. "A Plea for a Broader Concept of Nachträglichkeit." *Psychoanal Q.* 76 (2007): 1221–40.

Fassin, Didier, and Richard Rechtman. *The Empire of Trauma: An Inquiry into the Condition of Victimhood*. Princeton: Princeton University Press, 2009.

Felman, Shoshana, and Dori Laub. *Testimony: Crises of Witnessing in Literature, Psychoanalysis, and History*. New York: Routledge, 1992.

Ferenczi, Sándor. "Confusion of the Tongues Between the Adults and the Child (The Language of Tenderness and of Passion)." *Int. J. Psycho-Anal.* 30 (1949): 225–30.

Ferenczi, Sándor, Ernest Jones, Sigmund Freud, Ernst Simmel, and Karl Abraham. *Psycho-Analysis and the War Neuroses*. Vienna: The International Psycho-Analytical Press, 1921.

Ferraro, David. "Some Further Questions Prior to Any Possible Treatment of the Psychoses." *Psychoanalysis Lacan* 6 (2023): 69–76.

Fink, Bruce. *The Lacanian Subject: Between Language and Jouissance*. Princeton: Princeton University Press, 1995.

Flor, Rolf. "On the Very German-Ness of Freud's Trieb." In *Critical Essays on the Drive: Lacanian Theory and Practice*, edited by Dan Collins and Eve Watson, 43–52. The Lines of the Symbolic in Psychoanalysis Series. Abingdon, Oxon: Routledge, 2024.

Frege, Gottlob. *The Foundations of Arithmetic: A Logico-Mathematical Enquiry into the Concept of Number*. New York: Harper & Brothers, 1953.

Freud, Sigmund. "An Autobiographical Study." In *The Standard Edition of the Complete Psychological Works of Sigmund Freud*, XX:3–74. London: Hogarth Press, 1925.

———. "An Outline of Psycho-Analysis." In *The Standard Edition of the Complete Psychological Works of Sigmund Freud*, XXII:141–207. London: Hogarth Press, 1940.

———. "Beyond the Pleasure Principle." In *The Standard Edition of the Complete Psychological Works of Sigmund Freud*, XVIII:3–64. London: Hogarth Press, 1920.

———. "Civilisation and Its Discontents." In *The Standard Edition of the Complete Psychological Works of Sigmund Freud*, XXI:59–145. London: Hogarth Press, 1930.

———. "Constructions in Analysis." In *The Standard Edition of the Complete Psychological Works of Sigmund Freud*, XXIII:255–70. London: Hogarth Press, 1937.

———. "From the History of an Infantile Neurosis." In *The Standard Edition of the Complete Psychological Works of Sigmund Freud*, XVII:3–123. London: Hogarth Press, 1918.

———. "Hypnosis." In *The Standard Edition of the Complete Psychological Works of Sigmund Freud*, I:104–14. London: Hogarth Press, 1889a.

———. "Inhibitions, Symptoms and Anxiety." In *The Standard Edition of the Complete Psychological Works of Sigmund Freud*, XX:77–175. London: Hogarth Press, 1926.

———. "Instincts and Their Vicissitudes." In *The Standard Edition of the Complete Psychological Works of Sigmund Freud*, XIV:111–40. London: Hogarth Press, 1915a.

———. "Introductory Lectures on Psycho-Analysis." In *The Standard Edition of the Complete Psychological Works of Sigmund Freud*, Vol. XVI. London: Hogarth Press, 1916–1917.

———. "Moses and Monotheism." In *The Standard Edition of the Complete Psychological Works of Sigmund Freud*, XXIII:1–137. London: Hogarth Press, 1939.

———. "New Introductory Lectures on Psycho-Analysis." In *The Standard Edition of the Complete Psychological Works of Sigmund Freud*, XXII:3–182. London: Hogarth Press, 1933.

———. "On Narcissism: An Introduction." In *The Standard Edition Vol XIV*, XIV:69–102. London: Hogarth Press, 1914a.

———. "On the History of the Psychoanalytic Movement." In *The Standard Edition of the Complete Psychological Works of Sigmund Freud*, XIV:3–66. London: Hogarth Press, 1914b.

———. "Project for a Scientific Psychology." In *The Standard Edition Vol I*, I:281–397. London: Hogarth Press, 1950a.

———. "Repression." In *The Standard Edition of the Complete Psychological Works of Sigmund Freud*, V:143–58. London: Hogarth Press, 1915b.

———. "Review of August Forel's Hypnotism." In *The Standard Edition of the Complete Psychological Works of Sigmund Freud*, I:91–102. London: Hogarth Press, 1889b.

———. "Sexuality in the Aetiology of the Neuroses." In *The Standard Edition of the Complete Psychological Works of Sigmund Freud*, III:261–85. London: Hogarth Press, 1898.

———. "Sketches for the 'Preliminary Communication' of 1893." In *The Standard Edition of the Complete Psychological Works of Sigmund Freud*, I:147–54. London: Hogarth Press, 1940–1941.

———. *The Complete Letters of Sigmund Freud to Wilhelm Fliess 1887–1904*. Translated by Jeffrey M. Masson. Cambridge, Massachusetts: The Belkap Press of Harvard University Press, 1985.

———. "The Economic Problem of Masochism." In *The Standard Edition Vol XIX*, XIX:157–70. London: Hogarth Press, 1924.

———. "The Interpretation of Dreams (Second Part)." In *The Standard Edition of the Complete Psychological Works of Sigmund Freud*, V:339–627. London: Hogarth Press, 1900.

———. "The Neuroses of Defence (Extracts from the Fliess Papers: Draft K)." In *The Standard Edition of the Complete Psychological Works of Sigmund Freud*, I:220–28. London: Hogarth Press, 1950b.

———. "Three Essays on the Theory of Sexuality." In *The Standard Edition of the Complete Psychological Works of Sigmund Freud*, VII:125–245. London: Hogarth Press, 1905.

Freud, Sigmund, and Josef Breuer. "Studies on Hysteria." In *The Standard Edition of the Complete Psychological Works of Sigmund Freud*, Vol. II. London: Hogarth Press, 1895.

Gault, Jean-Louis. "Two Statuses of the Symptom: 'Let Us Turn to Finn Again.'" In *The Later Lacan: An Introduction*, edited by Véronique Voruz and Bogdan Wolf, 73–82. State of New York: Sunny Press, 2007.

Grigg, Russell. *Lacan, Language and Philosophy*. New York: State University of New York Press, 2008.

Guéguen, Pierre-Gilles. "Paradoxes of the Births of Transference." *Psychoanalytical Notebooks*, no. 17 (March 2008): 41–45.

Gueguen, Pierre-Gilles. "Transference: A Paradoxical Concept." *LC Express* 2, no. 12 (December 2014): 1–8.

Guéguen, Pierre-Gilles. "Who Is Mad and Who Is Not? On Differential Diagnosis in Psychoanalysis." *Culture/Clinic* 1 (2013): 66–85.

Harris, Oliver. *Lacan's Return to Anitiquity: Between Nature and the Gods*. Abingdon: Routledge, 2017.

Hawkins, Stephanie. "William James, Gustav Fechner, and Early Psychophysics." *Frontiers in Physiology* 2 (2011).

Horowitz, Mardi J. "Post Traumatic Stress Disorders." *Behavioral Sciences & the Law* 1, no. 3 (1983): 9–23.

House, Jonathan, and Julie Slotnick. "Apres-Coup in French Psychoanalysis: The Long Afterlife of Nachträglichkeit: The First Hundred Years, 1893 to 1993." *Psychoanalytic Review* 102, no. 5 (October 2015): 683–708.

Hynes, Samuel. *A War Imagined: The First World War and English Culture*. London: The Bodley Head Ltd, 1990.

Johnston, John. *The Allure of Machinic Life: Cybernetics, Artificial Life and the New AI*. Cambridge, Massachusetts: MIT Press, 2008.

Jones, Edgar, and Simon Wessely. "A Paradigm Shift in the Conceptualization of Psychological Trauma in the 20th Century." *Journal of Anxiety Disorders* 21, no. 2 (2007): 164–75.

Kardiner, Abram. *The Traumatic Neuroses of War*. Eastford, Connecticut: Martino Fine Books, 2012.

Kittler, Friedrich A. "The World of the Symbolic, A World of the Machine." In *Literature, Media, Information Systems*, edited by John Johnston, 130–46. London: Taylor & Francis Group, 1997.

Koyré, Alexandre. *From the Closed World to the Infinite Universe*. Baltimore: The Johns Hopkins University Press, 1957.

Lacan, Jacques. *Desire and Its Interpretation: The Seminar of Jacques Lacan Book VI*. Cambridge: Polity Press, 2019a.

———. "Joyce the Symptom." In *The Seminar of Jacques Lacan Book XXIII 1975–76: The Sinthome*, edited by Jacques-Alain Miller, 141–48. Cambridge: Polity Press, 2016a.

———. *Le Séminaire de Jacques Lacan: Livre XI Les Quatre Concepts Fondamentaux de La Psychanalyse 1964*. Paris: Éditions du Seuil, 1973.

———. "Position of the Unconscious." In *Écrits: The First Complete Edition in English*, 703–21. New York: W.W. Norton & Company, 2006a.

———. "Preface to the English Edition of Seminar XI." *The Lacanian Review*, no. 6 (2018): 22–27.

———. "Response to Jean Hyppolite's Commentary on Freud's 'Verneinung'." In *Écrits The First Complete Edition in Englsih*, translated by Bruce Fink, 318–33. New York: W.W. Norton & Company, 2006b.

———. "Science and Truth." In *Écrits: The First Complete Edition in English*, 726–45. New York: W.W. Norton & Company, 2006c.

———. *The Ethics of Psychoanalysis 1959–1960 The Seminar of Jacques Lacan Book VII*. London: Routledge, 1992.

———. *The Four Fundamental Concepts of Psycho-Analysis*. London: Penguin, 1979.

———. "The Function and Field of Speech and Language in Psychoanalysis." In *Écrits: The First Complete Edition in English*, 197–268. New York: W.W. Norton & Company, 2006d.

———. *The Object Relation: The Seminar of Jacques Lacan Book IV*. London: Polity Press, 2020.

———. *The Seminar of Jacques Lacan. Book II: The Ego in Freud's Theory and in the Technique of Psychoanalysis 1954–1955*. Cambridge: Cambridge University Press, 1988.

———. *The Seminar of Jacques Lacan Book IX 1961–62: Identification*. Translated by Cormac Gallagher. Dublin, 2002:

———. *The Seminar of Jacques Lacan Book V: Formations of the Unconscious*. Cambridge: Polity Press, 2017.

———. *The Seminar of Jacques Lacan: Book X: Anxiety 1962–1963*. Cambridge: Polity Press, 2014.

———. *The Seminar of Jacques Lacan Book XII Crucial Problems for Psychoanalysis*. Translated by Cormac Gallagher. Dublin: http://www.lacaninireland.com, 2011a.

———. *The Seminar of Jacques Lacan Book XIII The Object of Psychoanalysis*. Translated by Cormac Gallagher. Dublin, 2011b.

———. *The Seminar of Jacques Lacan Book XVIII 1971: On a Discourse That Might Not Be a Semblance*. Translated by Cormac Gallagher. Dublin, 2011c.

———. *The Seminar of Jacques Lacan Book XX 1972–1973: Encore*. Edited by Jacques-Alain Miller. New York: W.W. Norton & Company, 1999.

———. *The Seminar of Jacques Lacan: Book XXI: Les Non Dupres Errent: 1973–1974*. Translated by Cormac Gallagher. Dublin, 2010.

———. *The Seminar of Jacques Lacan Book XXII 1974–75: RSI*. Translated by Cormac Gallagher. Dublin, 2011d.

———. *The Sinthome: The Seminar of Jacques Lacan, Book XXIII*. Edited by Jacques-Alain Miller. Cambridge: Polity Press, 2016b.

———. "The Subversion of the Subject and the Dialectic of Desire in the Freudian Unconscious." In *Ecrits: The First Complete Edition in English*, 671–702. New York: W.W. Norton and Company, 2006e.

———. "The Third." *The Lacanian Review*, no. 7 (2019b): 83–109.

———. "There Are Four Discourses." *Culture/Clinic*, no. 1 (2013): 3–4.

Langer, Lawrence L. "Memory's Time: Chronology and Duration in Holocaust Testimonies." In *Admitting the Holocaust: Collected Essays*, 13–24. New York: Oxford University Press, 1995.

Laplanche, Jean. "Interview: Jean Laplanche Talks to Martin Stanton." In *Jean Laplanche: Seduction, Translation and the Drives*, translated by Martin Stanton, 3–18. London: Institute of Contemporary Arts, 1992.

———. *Life and Death in Psychoanalysis*. Baltimore: John Hopkins University Press, 1985.

———. *New Foundations for Psychoanalysis*. Oxford: Basil Blackwell, 1989.

———. "Notes on Afterwardsness." In *Essays on Otherness*, edited by John Fletcher, 260–65. Warwick Studies in European Philosophy. London: Routledge, 1999.

———. "Problématiques VI: Après-Coup." Translated by Jonathan House and Thurston. The Unconscious in Translation, 2017.

Laplanche, Jean, and Jean-Bertrand Pontalis. *The Language of Psychoanalysis*. London: Karnac Books, 1988.

Laurent, Eric. *Lost in Cognition: Psychoanalysis and the Cognitive Sciences*. London: Karnac, 2014.

Liddell, Henry George, and Robert Scott. *Liddell and Scott's Greek-English Lexicon: Abridged*. Simon Wallenberg Press, 2007.

Liu, Lydia H. *The Freudian Robot: Digital Media and the Future of the Unconscious*. Chicago: The University of Chicago Press, 2010.

Maleval, Jean-Claude. "Treatment of the Psychosis and Contemporary Psychoanalysis." In *Lacan on Madness: Madness, Yes You Can't*, edited by Patricia Gherovici and Manya Steinkoler, 99–111. Hove: Routledge, 2015.

Masson, Jeffrey M. *The Assault on Truth: Freud's Suppression of the Seduction Theory*. New York: Farrar, Strauss & Giroux, 1984.

Meretoja, Hanna, and Colin Davis. "Introduction to Literary Trauma Studies." In *The Routledge Companion to Literature and Trauma*, edited by Hanna Meretoja and Colin Davis, 1–8. Milton: Taylor and Francis, 2020.

Miller, Jacques-Alain. "Interpretation in Reverse." In *The Later Lacan: An Introduction*, edited by Véronique Voruz and Bogdan Wolf, 3–9. State of New York: Sunny Press, 2007.

———. "Is Feminine Jouissance Not Jouissance as Such?" *Lacanian Lnk*, no. 55/56 (2021): 34–51.

———. "Lacanian Biology and the Event of the Body." *Lacanian Lnk*, no. 18 (2001a): 6–29.

———. "Psychoanalysis, Its Place among the Sciences." *Psychoanalytical Notebooks*, no. 27 (September 2013): 9–19.

———. "Six Paradigms of Jouissance." *Psychoanalytical Notebooks*, no. 34 (December 2019): 11–77.

———. "Suture (Elements of the Logic of the Signifier)." *Screen* 18, no. 4 (December 1, 1977): 24–34.

———. "The Space of a Hallucination." *The Lacanian Review* 6, no. 6 (2018): 82–107.

———. "The Symptom and the Body Event." *Lacanian Lnk*, no. 19 (2001b): 4–47.

Moncayo, Raul. *Lalangue, Sinthome, Jouissance, and Nomination*. Abingdon: Routledge, 2017.

Murray, Jessica. "A Post-Colonial and Feminist Reading of Selected Testimonies to Trauma in Post-Liberation South Africa and Zimbabwe." *Journal of African Cultural Studies* 21, no. 1 (2009): 1–21.

Nadler, Steven. "Baruch Spinoza." In *The Stanford Encyclopedia of Philosophy*, edited by Edward N. Zalta, Summer 2022. Metaphysics Research Lab, Stanford University, 2022. https://plato.stanford.edu/archives/sum2022/entries/spinoza/.

Quinet, Antonio. "The Gaze as an Object." In *Reading Seminar XI: Lacan's Four Fundamental Concepts of Psychoanalysis*, edited by Richard Feldstein, Bruce Fink, and Maire Jaanus, 139–47. New York: State University of New York Press, 1995.

Rabeyron Thomas. "Psychoanalytic Psychotherapies and the Free Energy Principle." *Frontiers in Human Neuroscience* 16 (2022).

Reck, Erich. "Frege's Natural Numbers: Motivations and Modifications." In *Gottlob Frege: Critical Assessments of Leading Philosophers, Vol. III*, edited by Michael Beaney and Erich Reck, 270–301. Routledge, 2005.

Sauvagnat, François. "Fatherhood and Naming in J. Lacan's Works." The Symptom, 3, 2002. https://www.lacan.com/fathernamef.htm.

Shephard, Ben. *A War of Nerves*. London: Jonathan Cape, 2000.

Skriabine, Pierre. "Drive and Fantasy." *JCFAR*, no. 8 & 9 (1997): 28–44.

Spinoza, Benedict de. *Ethics*. London: Penguin Books, 1996.

Stevens, Alexandre. "The Bodily Effects of Language." In *NLS Congress*, 2020.

Strachey, James. "Some Technical Terms." In *The Standard Edition*, I:xxiii–xxvi. London: Hogarth Press, 1966.

Sütterlin, Nicole A. "History of Trauma Theory." In *The Routledge Companion to Literature and Trauma*, edited by Hanna Meretoja and Colin Davis, 11–22. Milton: Taylor and Francis, 2020.

Thomä, Helmut, and Neil Cheshire. "Freud's Nachträglichkeit and Strachey's 'Deferred Action': Trauma, Constructions and the Direction of Causality." *Int. R. Psycho-Anal.* 18 (1991): 407–27.

Vanderveken, Yves. "The Unconscious and the Brain: Nothing in Common." *The Lacanian Review*, no. 09 (2020): 198–213.

Verhaeghe, Paul. "A Combination That Has to Fail: New Patients, Old Therapists." *Eisteach (Dun Laoghaire)* 8, no. 4 (2008): 4–8.

———. "Causality in Science and Psychoanalysis." In *Lacan and Science*, edited by Jason Glynos and Yannis Stavrakakis, 119–45. London: Routledge, 2002.

———. "Subject and Body: Lacan's Struggle with the Real." In *Beyond Gender: From Subject to the Drive*, edited by Paul Verhaeghe, 65–97. New York: Other Press, 2001.

Verhaeghe, Paul, and Stijn Vanheule. "Actual Neurosis and PTSD: The Impact of the Other." *Psychoanalytic Psychology* 22, no. 4 (2005): 493–507.

Verhaeghe, Paul, Stijn Vanheule, and Ann De Rick. "Actual Neurosis as the Underlying Psychic Structure of Panic Disorder, Somatization, and Somatoform Disorder: An Integration of Freudian and Attachment Perspectives." *The Psychoanalytic Quarterly* 76, no. 4 (October 1, 2007): 1317–50.

Visser, Irene. "Decolonizing Trauma Theory: Retrospect and Prospects." *Humanities* 4, no. 2 (2015): 250–65.

Voruz, Véronique, and Bogdan Wolf, eds. *The Later Lacan: An Introduction*. New York: Suny Press, 2007.

Young, Allan. "W. H. R. Rivers and the War Neuroses." *Journal of the History of the Behavioral Sciences* 35, no. 4 (September 1, 1999): 359–78.

Zisser, Shirley. *Writing, Speech and Flesh in Lacanian Psychoanalysis: Of Unconscious Grammatology*. Abingdon, Oxon: Routledge, 2022.

Index

© The Author(s), under exclusive license to Springer Nature Switzerland AG 2025
L. Chapman, *Traumatic Neurosis Revisited*, The Palgrave Lacan Series,
https://doi.org/10.1007/978-3-031-89158-8

The manufacturer's authorised representative in the EU is Springer Nature Customer Service Centre GmbH, Europaplatz 3, 69115 Heidelberg, Germany. If you have any concerns regarding our products, please contact ProductSafety@springernature.com

Printed and bound by CPI Group (UK) Ltd, Croydon, CR0 4YY
01/10/2026
02225953-0007